Extreme Weight Loss Hypnosis Collection (4 in 1): Self-Hypnosis, Guided Meditations& Positive Affirmations For Rapid Fat Burning, Deep Sleep, Anxiety, Overthinking, Confidence

Extreme Weight Loss Hypnosis For Women: Guided Meditations, Affirmations& Hypnosis For Burning Fat Rapidly, Food Addiction& Emotional Eating& For Healthy Deep Sleep Habits

Extreme Weight Loss
A Hypnosis/Guided Meditation series

In this 5-hour series, we explore extreme weight loss, naturally, through guided hypnosis and meditation.

This audiobook will include a series of Hypnotherapy sessions, guided meditations and affirmations, that will transform the hearts and minds of listeners who are desperately seeking ways to lose weight.

All sessions are original content, written by a qualified Hypnotherapist with extensive experience in helping people achieve their personal life goals naturally.

The Sessions

The sessions will unfold as follows:

Introduction:.. 5

Session 1: Extreme Weight Loss Mindset 7

Session 2: Extreme Weight Loss Sleep Hypnosis 15

Session 3: Extreme Weight Loss Overcome Food Addiction 23

Session 4: Extreme Weight Loss No More Emotional Eating 31

Session 5: Extreme Weight loss Burn Fat Rapidly...................................... 37

Bonus Session: Extreme Weight Loss Affirmations.................................... 44

Introduction:

About this Audiobook.

Who this audiobook is suitable for What results you can expect How to use this content.

Session 1. Extreme Weight Loss: Mindset

Overview:

A 45-min Hypnosis session.

This session will introduce mental conditioning that will create an extreme weight loss mindset for the listener. The session will include an introduction to hypnosis, a relaxing induction, deepener and hypnotic suggestions. **Session 2. Extreme Weight Loss: Improved Sleep**

Overview:

A 45-min Hypnosis session.

This deep sleep hypnosis is written to encourage the listener to fall asleep. This session will include a deep relaxation induction, hypnotic suggestions for cell regeneration, appetite reset, improved sleeping patterns and of course extreme weight loss.

Session 3. Extreme Weight Loss: Overcome food addiction

Overview:
A 60-min Hypnosis session.
During this hypnosis session, the listener will be guided to explore the triggers that have caused unhealthy eating habits, including takeout, and sugary food. The hypnotic suggestions will reprogram these triggers, replacing them with healthy alternative actions such as exercise, meditation, yoga and eating healthy foods. **Session 4. Extreme Weight Loss: No more emotional eating**

Overview:

A 30-min Hypnosis session.
This session will address the patterns of emotional eating that is a deep-rooted response to the stressors of life, most likely created during childhood. The listener will experience a relaxing induction, deep deepener, allowing them to reset their emotional responses to a healthy alternative, in place of eating.

Session 5. Extreme weight loss: Burn fat rapidly

Overview:

A 45-min Hypnosis session.

This session will program the mind to seek ways to burn fat rapidly, daily. With a deep relaxation induction and deepener, the hypnotic suggestions included are designed to reprogram any deep-set beliefs around exercise and fat-burning activity.

Session 6. Extreme Weight Loss: Affirmations

A 30-min Subliminal affirmation session.

This session will include a series of powerful present moment affirmations that will reinforce the reprogramming of the previous hypnotic sessions.

Conclusion

Thank you for listening

Find more help @_____

Session 1: Extreme Weight Loss Mindset

Overview: This session will introduce mental conditioning that will create an extreme weight loss mindset for the listener. The session will include an introduction to hypnosis, a relaxing induction, deepener and hypnotic suggestions.

Time: 45-minutes

[Reader Notes]

- Read the following script at a steady pace, taking your time to guide the listener with your voice.
- Allow long comfortable pauses in between passages, that you are happy with, and follow the key set out below to allow longer pauses.

[Pause Key]

/ Short pause: Reader pauses for 10 seconds

// Medium pause: Reader pauses for 20 seconds

/// Long pause: Reader pauses for 30 seconds

Hello and welcome to this powerful hypnotic session, from _____ *[Script Begins]*

Welcome to the first session in the Extreme Weight Loss series.

Congratulations on making the decision to start your Extreme Weight Loss journey! If you have tried liver cleansing, apple cider vinegar, vibrating machines, portion size and paleo, then you have finally arrived at the right place.

This hypnosis audio will allow your subconscious mind to be reprogrammed with the secret formula that creates the extreme weight loss mindset.... and all you have to do is relax and breathe. My name is _____ and I'll be your guide during this experience.

Let's be honest for a second, we live in a world where body image is at the forefront of all of our minds, and as a result we are all bombarded with new weight loss trends that are popping up faster than you can say Atkins! The sad truth is, that 95 % of people who try to lose weight by starting on the outside, put it all back on, plus more, within less than a year!. The question is why?

Here at Extreme Weight Loss, we have done the research, and studied the studies, so that you can finally achieve weight loss success. You see the key factor in successful weight loss and weight maintenance moving forward is simply changing your mind.

The brain determines why, how and where body fat is stored. The brain drives our metabolism, hunger, food choices, discipline and inspiration to exercise, or not and hormone production. The good news is that you can alter the brain, by changing your mind, it really is that simple. We call this creating a new mindset. The mind is where we get to create a new set of beliefs, programs and instructions that will change the chemistry, hormone, metabolism, hunger and discipline in the brain.

So, it's time to let go of the anxiety, stress, diet plan, calorie counter and take a deep breath, relax and let your mind do the work.

/

As you make yourself comfortable, I want you to know that Hypnosis is not mind control, you will remain in full control throughout this audiobook and whenever you want to stop for whatever reason, you can simply hit pause. All hypnosis is self hypnosis and the idea behind the Extreme Weight Loss series is that you will reprogram your mind, with my help, and create the life you deserve.

Find a comfortable position, where you can relax fully with your head and body supported. If you are sitting in a chair then you can allow your head to nod forward, or fall back against the headrest.

//

Take a long deep breath, fill up your lungs and hold it for a second. Now when you exhale,

And now as you continue to breathe nice and deeply allow your attention to float up towards your mind where we will begin the process of relaxing you nice and deeply while installing the extreme weight loss mindset…..

and taking a nice deep breath in through the nose and as you allow your mind to drift to a
new identity…. One where you have achieved extreme weight loss….. I would like you to count down from 100 - 0… taking you deep into a relaxed state…. After all, that is all that hypnosis is …. Deep relaxation…. Where you can forget all of your worries… all of your concerns and most importantly…. You can leave all of the stress of losing weight behind you……

Let's begin counting now……100… and you can count down with me….99….98….97….96….95…..94….93….92….91….

90…. excellent and keep counting now in your mind….

89…88…87…. allowing you to relax completely ….deeply with ease…. And as you continue to count slowly and deliberately… I would like you to listen to my voice…. And as you listen to my voice… continue counting deeper and deeper…

///

as you exhale just allow your entire body to relax and let go of any tension that you may be holding onto as you know all change starts in the mind and today ……through this very special hypnotic session you will be given a mindset transplant…. That's right, a mindset transplant…. Where your old mindset will be replaced with a new mindset…. The mindset of extreme weight loss…. And once you have this mindset losing extreme amounts of weight will be so easy for you…. It will be as easy as clicking your fingers or clapping your hands….

Keep counting down….. and as you count ….continue breathing nice and deeply

//

And let yourself relax. Get rid of that surface tension in your body, let your shoulders relax. It's ok to just relax today.

Now put your awareness on your eyelids. You know that you can relax those eyes beautifully… and as you relax them you can start to see an image in your mind's eye of the body you so greatly desire for yourself…. After all, that is the reason you are here today and listening to my voice isn't it?...... for the extreme weight loss mindset you have always desired…..

You know that you can relax those eyes so deeply, that as long as you choose not to remove that relaxation, those eyelids just won't work… And when you know that you've done that, hold on to that relaxation, give them a good test, make sure they won't work…

And notice how good it feels. Test them hard, it's ok.

///

Stop testing… now let yourself relax even more…. That quality of relaxation you are allowing in your eyes is the quality of relaxation I'd like you to let yourself have throughout your entire body…

So take that same quality, bring it up to the top of your head… And send it down through your body from the top of your head to the tip of your toes. Let go of every muscle. Let go of every nerve. Let go of every fibre... And let yourself drift much, deeper, relaxed. You got it.... And I want you to know that the more you relax the easier it will be for your subconscious mind to accept the secret to the extreme weight loss mindset......

Now let's really deepen this state. In a moment I'll ask you to open and close your eyes. When you close your eyes, send a wave of relaxation through your body, so very quickly, you'll allow this physical part of you to relax...

/

And from this moment on every breath... each and every breath that you exhale relaxes you more and more... from this moment on each and every breath that you exhale helps you to receive the secrets of the extreme weight loss mindset with your unconscious mind and close down the doubts and concerns of your conscious mind........ and as you listen to my voice it helps you to be just more and more calm...

and from this moment on doing those things which you know inside your mind will help you to reach your ideal weight and achieve your ideal body... doing those things feels completely normal... and completely natural for you in every way possible... and this suggestion and this idea now grows strong inside your mind... this suggestion and this idea becomes more and more real for you... not because I say so... but because it's the suggestion that you want in your life... and because it's the suggestion that you do want in your life... it does now mean that doing those things which you know inside your mind will help you to achieve the extreme weight loss mindset .....and as a result, you reach your ideal weight... and stay there.....and it will feel easy and completely natural for you in every way possible...

and as you now continue to relax physically... and as you now continue to relax mentally just more and more with every breath... your wonderful unconscious mind... the part of your mind that knows everything about you... the part of your mind that can easily and naturally guide you towards your ideal weight... now begins to become open... open to the wonderful suggestions that you're going to receive today...

//

so continue relaxing more and more now with every breath... and as you continue to relax just more and more with every breath I'm going to share with you the four secrets to an extreme weight loss mindset ..... and that very first secret to an extreme weight loss mindset is to know exactly what it is that you do want... far too many people when they think about losing weight... and they think about the reasons why they want to lose weight... far too many people focus on the negative aspects... people might think to themselves that they don't want to be overweight anymore... they don't want to be unhealthy... don't want to be in such and such a size of clothing... it's important with regards to your weight that you know... and you focus on the reasons why you want to be a certain size... by focusing on the reasons why... you'll stay completely motivated... and you'll stay determined...

so begin now to think... think in your mind the reasons why you want to achieve an extreme weight loss mindset and become such and such a size... such and such a weight... is it for that party... that wedding you may have coming up... is it to be able to go into that clothes department and to choose those clothes that you want to wear... do you want to be a certain size... a certain weight... in order to be healthier... to feel fitter in yourself... or is it in order to feel and to be more confident... more comfortable in yourself... just spend a few moments now thinking about the reasons why you want to be a certain size... a certain weight... think about these reasons in the positive sense...

it's important that when you're striving for a goal you focus on the reasons why... and those reasons why have to be more than just a number... more than just a size... if you focus just on a number... if you focus just on a size then you might feel motivated at first... but that motivation will drain away... you want to be such and such a size... such and such a weight for the things that being such a size... such a weight is going to give you... and by focusing on those wonderful positive benefits you'll stay motivated... you'll stay determined... and you'll stay completely focused... spend a few moments now thinking about those reasons why... and I'll give you a few moments as you do so...

///

The reasons why you want to have an extreme weight loss mindset is so you can..... achieve such a size... such a weight... and that's the first secret to your weight loss success... knowing exactly what it is you want... but knowing what you want in the positive sense...

The second secret of having an extreme weight loss mindset is to use your imagination... imagine yourself being at that weight... imagine yourself wearing that beach outfit....... Or those clothes... imagine yourself being and feeling confident... because one of the things about your imagination is every time you imagine something you're actually giving your unconscious mind that blueprint of how you want to be... and then once your unconscious mind has got that positive blueprint of how you want to be... your unconscious mind will then begin to move you towards that blueprint... and losing weight then will just seem easy and completely natural in every way possible...

//

as I said your imagination to your unconscious mind is real... your unconscious mind doesn't know the difference between something real and something imagined... so by imagining yourself how you want to be... imagining yourself wearing those clothes... imagining yourself being and feeling confident... you then begin to send the idea to your unconscious mind that you truly are at the weight you want to be... and then your unconscious mind begins to follow this blueprint... your unconscious mind then begins to move you towards your ideal weight...

so let's now use your imagination… I want you now to imagine yourself at your ideal weight… imagine yourself may be putting on an item of clothing… looking at yourself in the mirror… or maybe imagine other people commenting on how good you look… spend a few moments and actually imagine yourself being at your ideal weight… and I'll give you a few moments as you do so…

and again you can just keep continuing to use your imagination in this wonderful positive manner… imagining yourself being at your ideal weight… beginning then to give your unconscious mind that wonderful positive blueprint… and that's the second secret of having an extreme weight loss mindset ….
///

The third secret of the extreme weight loss mindset is to ensure that your self talk… the things that you say to yourself… the things that you say to other people… match the outcomes that you're striving for… your self-talk is important… in a sense, you can think of your self talk… you can think of yourself as having two aspects… that first aspect of yourself is the thinker… everybody thinks… and there's no limit to what you can think… you can think you're overweight… you can think that you have a sweet tooth… you can think that you're addicted to fatty foods… there's no limit to what you can think… but it's important what you do think matches the outcomes that you're striving for… making sure that your thoughts are positive… telling yourself that you're in control of food… telling yourself that you exercise on a regular basis… it's important that the things that you do tell yourself on a regular basis are positive and match those outcomes that you're striving for… and as I said everybody thinks… there is a thinker inside you…

and another aspect that you also have inside of you is an aspect called the prover… and that proving part of you only has one job… and that's to prove what you think to be true… so if you have those thoughts that you have a sweet tooth the prover in you will then just prove to you that you do have a sweet tooth… and you will have a sweet tooth… but if you start to have those wonderful positive thoughts that you are in complete control of food… the prover in you will then just prove to you that you are in complete control of food… and you will be in complete control of food…

so from this moment on your thoughts do now just become more and more positive each and every day… and that's the third secret of the powerful extreme weight loss mindset… ensuring that your self-talk is positive… ensuring that your self-talk matches the outcomes that you're striving for…

///

The fourth and final secret of the extreme weight loss mindset is each and every day doing those things which you know inside your mind will move you towards your ideal weight… think about losing weight very much like playing a board game… and you might think well what does a board game and losing weight have in common… but these two things have a lot in common… because just like playing a board game you know what you want… you know what size you want to be… you know what weight you want to be… and just like playing a board you want to win... you want to get to the end... and you then roll the dice... the dice might land on number four... and you move those four spaces forward... maybe like one of those weeks during which your weight does decrease... you're moving towards your goal... you're moving towards your ideal weight... you feel good in yourself... you feel motivated... you feel confident... and you have that strong belief that you're going to reach your target...

you then roll the dice again and this time it lands on three and again you move another three spaces forward... another three spaces closer towards where you want to be... again you feel good... you feel motivated... you feel confident... and that belief that you're going to reach your ideal weight grows even stronger... you then roll the dice again... this time it might land on number two... and you move two spaces forward... again you feel good because you're moving towards your goal... but as you look down you realise that you've landed on a square that says miss a turn... in a sense moving towards your dream body can be quite similar to landing on one of these squares that says miss a turn... yes you might have one of those weeks where your weight stays the same...

and if you get one of those weeks... or even a couple of weeks where your weight stays the same... it's important that you focus on the big picture... it's important that you focus on how far you've travelled... how much closer you are towards your goal... not allowing that little set back to knock you off course... staying motivated... staying completely determined...

... and you then roll the dice again... it lands on four and again you're starting to make progress... again moving once again towards your ideal weight... towards where you want to be... you soon forget about that time when you missed a turn... and you feel good because you feel closer to where you want to be... you then roll the dice again... maybe this time it lands on five and you move five spaces forward... but this time you might land on a square that says go back two spaces... again you feel annoyed because you've had to go back two spaces... and again when moving towards your ideal... yes you may have one of those weeks... or a couple of those weeks during which your weight increases a little bit... and if that does happen to you... it's important that you stay focused... it's important that you keep that goal at the forefront of your mind...

because if you keep that goal in the forefront of your mind... you'll overcome this and any other set back... you'll continue the journey... you'll keep rolling that dice... moving forward... being focused on the goal... and you'll then reach that goal... you'll feel good in yourself... you'll feel that wonderful sense of achievement... you'll feel good knowing that yes along the way you may have had some setbacks... but you stayed motivated... you stayed determined... you stayed completely focused... and that's the fourth step to keeping yourself motivated... to keep doing those things which you know will help you to reach your ideal weight... to stay motivated during those setbacks... to keep your eyes on that goal...

///

Those are the four keys to the extreme weight loss mindset transplant that has now taken place in your mind... the first real secret... knowing what you want... but knowing what you want in the positive sense... the second secret... using your powerful imagination... imagining yourself being at your ideal weight... the third secret... ensuring that your self talk... ensuring what you're saying to yourself is matching those outcomes that you want in your life... and the fourth and final secret is to keep doing those things which you know inside your mind will help you to reach your ideal weight as your new extreme weight loss mindset kicks in and starts to take effect.... to keep doing those things even during those weeks when you have a setback... to stay focused on the goal... these are the four secrets to real extreme weight loss ...

and don't dismiss these secrets because they seem too easy... because the easy things in life are the most complex... if you think about it there are twenty-six letters in the alphabet... but those twenty-six simple letters make a dictionary of words... and that dictionary of words make an infinite number of sentence combinations... and there was once a time when you couldn't even put three simple letters together... c... a... t... to spell cat... whereas you now know... you can do this without even thinking about it...

the easy things in life are the most complex... if you think about it there are ten digits... one to nine and zero... but these ten simple digits make an infinite number of numbers... and there was once a time when you couldn't even put three simple numbers together... one... two... three... were as now you can do that without even thinking about it... the easy things in life are the most complex and these four simple secrets to weight loss success do and will create wonderful positive change in you... and these suggestions and these ideas now just become more and more clear for you... every single day...

And in a few moments, I am going to bring this session to a close...and when I do you will awaken feeling optimistic and energised about your new extreme weight loss mindset....

And I am going to count from 0 - 3 and on 3 you will open your eyes and it will be as if you were never in a hypnotic state... and you will accept and believe every suggestion that you heard during this hypnosis session...

And 1... ... 2... 3 and eyes open and welcome back!

Thank you for listening to this powerful hypnotic experience...... remember, the results will continue to develop long after this session has finished. And each time you listen, the results get progressively deeper.

Session 2: Extreme Weight Loss Sleep Hypnosis

Overview: This deep sleep hypnosis is written to encourage the listener to fall asleep.
This session will include a deep relaxation induction, hypnotic suggestions for cell regeneration, appetite reset, improved sleeping patterns and of course extreme weight loss.

Time: 45-minutes

[Reader Notes]

- Read the following script at a steady pace, taking your time to guide the listener with your voice.
- Allow long comfortable pauses in between passages, that you are happy with, and follow the key set out below to allow longer pauses.

[Pause Key]

/ Short pause: Reader pauses for 10 seconds

// Medium pause: Reader pauses for 20 seconds

/// Long pause: Reader pauses for 30 seconds

Hello and welcome to this powerful hypnotic session, from _____

[Script Begins]

As you embark on your extreme weight loss journey, there is a really important lifestyle change that supports weight loss immensely. Getting a regular good night's sleep. Sleep deprivation increases the levels of all of the hormones that create mouth hunger and sugar cravings. As if that wasn't enough, being tired also drives us to eat as a way of giving us the energy we need to get through the day.

The good news is, this hypnosis audio will guide you into a state of relaxation and deep sleep, even if you are struggling with insomnia. By enjoying a good night's sleep you increase the impact of any weight loss strategies you might be using including this series, The Extreme Weight Loss series.

Make yourself comfortable in bed, fluff your pillows and remember, as soona s your head hits the pillow, you will become open to the idea of having a good night's sleep as part of your weight loss journey…. My name is _____ and I'll be your guide during this experience.

//

To begin it is very easy, all you have to do is listen to my voice and go with me as we relax into a calming sense of ease…

Allow the sense of relaxation to deepen as you enter into a state of peacefulness …

Where we are going now there's no need to strive, no need to try or put any effort into thinking consciously… in fact all you have to do is breathe….

Breathing deeply helps you relax better…Relaxing more fully helps you to reduce stress and cortisol…. Helping you to lose weight at the same time….. In fact, breathing deeply helps to restore all the systems and functions in your body… to their perfect settings… keeping your mind and body balanced in a state that we call homeostasis.

Let your breath be deep and slow. Relax…and continue to relax… deeper and deeper… as you breathe in more…fresh, pure oxygen. Breathe in very fully… and notice yourself relaxing… more and more …with each breath.

//

As we begin this session your full co-operation is needed to relax the body and the mind by taking several deep breaths and releasing any tension or concerns as you drift into the deep state of hypnosis.

/

Now… I want you to add counting to your breathing like this.

Breathe in …3…4…5…6. Hold…2…3…Breathe out…3…4…5….6….

Breathe in…3…4…5…6… Hold 2…3…Breathe out…3…4…5…6….

Breathe in …3…4…5…6…. Hold…2…3… Breathe out…3…4…5….6….

Breathe in…3…4…5…6… Hold 2…3…Breathe out… 3…4…5…6….

Continue this breathing rhythm with the 6-3-6 count for at least ten times while I continue to talk to you. As you continue to breathe deeply, you send stress-reducing oxygen to all the cells,.. muscles, ..bones, ..organs …and systems of your body.

//

As you notice the relaxation beginning to ease around and through your entire body, surrender to it… there is no need to fight or resist… let go and become relaxed….

Close your eyes … take a deep breath … and as you exhale, imagine the number 3 in front of you … See it as if it were projected on a screen, slightly above your eye level, approximately 5 to 6 feet away from your head … Take a second deep breath … and as you exhale imagine the number 2 on that screen … Even with your eyes closed try to feel the eye strain from looking upward as if you are looking through your eyelids at that screen … Take a third deep breath … hold it for a few seconds … and as you exhale imagine the number 1 on that screen … allowing yourself to let go completely, and relax …

To relax even deeper, I'd like you to imagine the numbers 10, all the way down to 1 … on the screen, as you hear them spoken … taking your time … allowing yourself to relax twice as deep, with each number that you imagine … When you get to the number 1 … you will be in the Alpha Brainwave State… which is a state where the subconscious mind is very receptive and open to suggestion …

Now let's begin with …

10 … Allow yourself to relax completely …

9 … Just letting go …

8 … Imagine the number as you relax twice as deep …

7 … See it as clearly as you can, just let go …

6 … All the way down deep …

5 … Deeper and deeper, taking your time …

4 … Allowing all outside sounds to fade away completely …

3 … Just imagine the number and let yourself go …

2 … Deeper and deep … and finally

1 … Deep … deep … relaxation…

You are now in a state of relaxation where you are more open to suggestions … In this relaxed state, your mind can expand … and is much more receptive and sensitive than in any other state … So just allow yourself to continue to relax … and enjoy this comfortable feeling …

As I give you the following suggestions I'd like you to imagine everything I say in your mind... Imagine yourself as if you were watching yourself on a movie screen and you can change the scene magically to anything you like. Just use your imagination and have fun with it... as you continue to hear and focus on my words...

//

Now...as you continue to focus on the screen...I want you to notice a colour of your choice...a calming relaxing colour...coming in through the top of your head as you inhale..... See this relaxing colour come in through the top of your head ...and gradually fill every cell in your body...Notice as this relaxing colour filters down from the top of your head... through your face and neck...down into your shoulders and arms..relaxing, soothing...through your chest and pelvic region...soothing and relaxing all your internal organs...down through your hips, thighs and knees... relaxing any tightness or inflexibility...relaxing deeper....down into your calves...and finally into your ankles, feet... and out through your toes....taking all toxins and other negative energies that were in your body...out...

Notice that you are now standing at the top of some steps...maybe wooden steps, maybe stone...any steps that you imagine are fine.

///

Just see yourself standing at the top of ten steps...leading down to the ocean. It is a brilliant summer day... as you stand at the top of these steps. Notice the beautiful, blue sky above you... and the birds singing cheerfully...Notice how wonderful the day is...Notice how you are feeling...

As you begin to descend these steps, going down from 10 down to 1, you will gradually go deeper and deeper into hypnosis... And when you get down to the bottom, you will be perfectly relaxed, and calm at a very deep level of consciousness, a level where you KNOW you can reprogram your body and mind effortlessly...

So begin now to descend these steps... 10 ....going down now, easily 9 ....perfectly peaceful and calm 8 ....totally tranquil 7 ....deeper and deeper 6 ....even deeper still 5 ....very relaxed now 4 ....relaxing even more 3 ....very serene now 2 ....almost there 1 ....totally relaxed and centred now.

Now...as you step off gently...into the warm, summer sand...you feel more at peace and relaxed than ever before in your entire life...

//

Notice yourself walking towards the beach...Notice the feel of the sand under your feet...the ocean breeze in your hair, and the sun on your shoulders. Notice all the sensations around you. Very relaxed and at ease.

Now...notice a bag in front of you, directly in your path...It might be a paper grocery bag, or maybe a large black plastic bag ... Any kind of bag you imagine is just fine.

Just walk over and pick it up. As you pick up the bag...you become aware that there are things you wish to discard from your life. They might be sweet treats that are preventing you from losing weight…. Or worries about weight gain and body image that are keeping you awake at night….. Whatever these stressful thoughts and feelings are that may have carried around ……about your weight or how you look and feel….it's time to let them go by placing them in the bag…..

You might wish to discard old beliefs that no longer serve you or negative imprints that keep you from losing weight and getting a good night's sleep…… Perhaps you need to let go of responsibilities that are not really yours and are holding you back……. Any negative or harmful thoughts, impressions, beliefs, feelings, or experiences can now be discarded into the bag easily, released effortlessly.

/

See yourself removing them now...and as you do...notice that you are feeling better. Perhaps you feel lighter as if a burden has been lifted from your shoulders.

Whatever improvement you feel is fine. Just allow yourself to soak up this wonderful new feeling, along with the summer sun. Breathe in deeply and absorb this new and improved feeling throughout your body...

And know that this new feeling will grow stronger every time you visit this relaxing place in your mind. And once you have your bag completely full... of all the negatives you wish to discard...pick it up ...and toss it as far out into the ocean...as far as you can throw it...And...as it floats away …. Far out to sea….. You watch it as it eventually begins to sink….. And as it sinks…..you realize that those negatives you discarded will never affect you again...You have now released them permanently...You are now free to reshape your life and body in any way that you want... and you know now that a good night's sleep is an essential part of your extreme weight loss journey….

//

See yourself on the movie screen exactly as you want to be...relaxed, calm and functioning well in every way...happy, healthy, vibrantly alive, loved, loving and successful...truly fulfilled and living in peace and tranquillity with all those around you.

And, as the last of your released stressors sink to the bottom of the ocean, continue your pleasant walk along the beach…

As you walk along the beach you come across a large comfortable lounger… with an umbrella for shade and a side table with a cool glass of fresh water waiting for you….

As you make yourself comfortable in the lounge…. You lie back …. Take a sip of the water…… and relax….. Relaxing deeper and deeper as the session goes on…..

And as you lay here beneath the parasol…. Shielding you from the sun….. You become drowsy…. Sleepy and drowsy….. And before you know it…. You begin to nod off……

///

And as you fall into a deep restful sleep you become even more open to the positive suggestions that I have for you about your extreme weight loss journey… in fact your unconscious mind is so open and so receptive to everything I have to say now…. That it becomes a relaxing and restful experience listening to my voice…

And I want you to know that you are in control of your body and your mind…. And when you need to sleep and rest your body and mind… you can do so automatically…. In fact, as soon as you make the decision to go to sleep as soon as your head hit the pillow… you find yourself drifting off into a deep regenerating sleep with ease……

and you realize that sleep is essential for extreme weight loss… and knowing this you realize that you must take control of your mind and body when it comes to sleep….. And because you know that your thoughts create your reality… you protect the thoughts that allow you to rest in a timely manner and you reject the thoughts that tell you to stay up and watch TV … and you reject the negative thoughts that linger in your mind when it's time for sleep… You focus only on good things… Positive thoughts …

///

You are weight loss-oriented… You know it is important to do everything that helps you to lose weight fast…. Including quality sleep… Now I'd like you to imagine that you already succeeded in attaining your weight loss… In fact, let's have some fun with it… I'd like you to imagine yourself sitting in a movie theatre all by yourself watching yourself on a movie screen right in front of you as an actor in a movie you're creating with your own mind… You're the director and whatever you imagine actually happens on the screen… Don't worry you'll be completely safe and comfortable…

Imagine the end result of your weight loss… Imagine it has already happened in all its detail… Have fun with it and create it just the way you want it to be…

Now it's time to break it down step by step… Think about what it took to achieve this weight loss starting from when you first thought of it? What are the steps you'll need to take to make it happen? What needs to come together? What do you have to consider? Healthy food… plenty of exercise… drink lots of water… get lots of sleep…..

Imagining your completed weight loss in front of you now gives you the ability to figure out how to make it happen… Think about the step-by-step process of what you have to do… Take some time doing this and make sure you include every small detail that contributed to your extreme weight loss journey….

///

Realize that since you created your weight loss in your mind that you CAN accomplish it… What your mind can conceive it can achieve… Everything that has ever been created was first created as a thought… just as you're doing here. This is your "blueprint" and now you only have to follow the steps in your blueprint to create your weight loss.

You can do it… You are a creative person… You have the abilities to accomplish your task… and the knowledge you have from your blueprint will help you to get anything together you may need that you might not already have at your disposal.

Allow yourself to commit all the details of your weight loss blueprint to memory. Memorize all the details so when you open your eyes at the end of this session you'll have them fresh and clear in your mind for retrieval… right at your fingertips.

/

You have succeeded… You obtained your weight loss in your mind… Now you can go out and create it in reality… You are motivated… Energized… and anxious to move forward in all that you do… You look forward to the opportunity and new challenges… You are self-driven … and eager to live your new focus of positive thinking and successful living…

/

You are successful … You act and think as someone who has already experienced extreme weight loss…. As somebody who sleeps at least 8-hours every night…. You act and behave like the person you want to be… You realize that you create your own reality according to your focus … Therefore you remain focussed on positive things… You deserve weight loss success… It is your right to lose weight and this includes having a good night's sleep every single night….. You are comfortable with your new bedtime routine…. You are even more comfortable with your lifestyle…. You expect to be in full control of your body and mind at all times and it is so…..

//

You welcome change with a smile... You realize that you are very flexible and able to change when change is required...

When you wake up tomorrow morning, ... you will feel different... you will feel fresh... well rested and you will have a new belief... your new belief will be that you are committed to sleeping well every night as a part of your weight loss journey... you will believe that you are committed to weight loss and in fact everything in your life is geared towards extreme weight loss....be able to recall easily and completely ...all the information you gathered from this session... to help you continue the process of enjoying deep restful sleep and extreme weight loss.... That's right, good quality sleep of at least 8-hours a night is a part of your extreme weight loss success story....

In the next few hours, days or weeks, any restrictions, tightness or inflexibility that was uncovered and is not beneficial for you will be easily released...

You now understand clearly that negative emotions or feelings sometimes become stuck in the mind or the body and by coming to this relaxing place, ...as often as you like... you can encourage deep relaxation of the body, mind and all you have to do... is relax and breathe deeply... and enjoy healing and regenerating sleep... every night....

You really ARE in charge of your own life, through the power of hypnosis and connecting with the subconscious mind!

The more you use hypnosis ...the easier it will be to fall asleep and enjoy a good quality night's sleep.....

Every time you listen to this session, you will go more deeply, more quickly...and you will gain more insights improving the quality of your sleep and losing even more weight as a result....

Sleep well!

Session 3: Extreme Weight Loss Overcome Food Addiction

Overview: During this hypnosis session, the listener will be given a new mind program that will override the existing addiction to food programming that has caused weight gain and unhealthy eating habits, in their life. The deep hypnotic suggestions will reprogram the mind, replacing old patterns of behaviour with healthy alternative actions such as exercise, meditation, yoga and eating healthy foods.

Time: 60-minutes

[Reader Notes]

- Read the following script at a steady pace, taking your time to guide the listener with your voice.
- Allow long comfortable pauses in between passages, that you are happy with, and follow the key set out below to allow longer pauses.

[Pause Key]

/ Short pause: Reader pauses for 10 seconds

// Medium pause: Reader pauses for 20 seconds

/// Long pause: Reader pauses for 30 seconds

Hello and welcome to this powerful hypnotic session, from _____

[Script Begins]

Hello and welcome to this powerful hypnotic session, brought to you by_____

Food addiction! Just like any other addiction, it creeps up over time, becoming a way to suppress feelings, destress, and medicate the pains and difficulties that life can often bring. Food has become complicated in recent decades, with companies combining fat and sugar to create addictive food products such as cakes, cookies and donuts. Takeaways and fast food are pumped full of chemicals that create cravings as strong as cocaine cravings, and sugar, the most addictive substance on earth, is wrapped up in bright and colourful packaging, that tricks the brain into thinking it is safe to eat.

So, how do you overcome food addiction? While it's not easy, just like any other addiction, the change MUST start in the mind. Thankfully, our brains are plastic and with just a few sessions like this one, you can reprogram the neural pathways that cause you to crave addictive foods, and instead replace those urges and desires with healthy foods, or activities that will add to your extreme weight loss journey.

Make yourself nie and comfortable, preferably sitting up as we begin this powerful hypnosis session, that will allow you to overcome your deep desire for overeating and indulging in addictive foods. My name is _____ and I'll be your guide during this experience.

/

As this hypnosis session begins there is nothing for you to do except listen to my voice as I guide you into a deep state of relaxation where your conscious mind sleeps and your unconscious mind takes over... and all you need to do to achieve this is breathe.... Nice and deeply...

And just notice how your body moves as you breathe nice and deeply... allowing each breath to fill the entire body... calming the mind and releasing any tightness or tension that may be present in the body...

/

Simply make yourself comfortable in the place you have chosen and close your eyes............. this is your time for yourself... empty your mind of all thoughts but listen to the sound of my voice... which will help you to relax...the sound of my voice... will help you to relax.

Your mind may wander...but the sound of my voice will travel with you ... all the time helping you............. to relax.................remember why you are here... to let go of your food addiction ... to create a healthy way of eating and living your life, and most importantly to experience extreme weight loss by eating only healthy, clean, small portions of food, even when you are triggered by past trauma or the stress of daily life.

As you listen to my voice you are totally ready to relax.... Notice now, the rate of your breathing.......... and begin to slow it down............... and every time you breathe out you can also begin to relax even more............ every time you breathe out..........you can begin to let go of any physical tension in any part of your body................so while you............... continue to slow down and deepen your breathing.................. you can also begin to.............. relax from the top of your head all the way down............... you will relax from the top of the head down............and as you relax from the top of the head down.... I will count down from 10 to 0....

//

So... starting with the crown of your head....I would like you to imagine you can relax the muscles in your scalp................10...... .... and then let go of the muscles in your forehead.............9.......and now your eyebrows...... 8....................and allow your eyelids to remain comfortably closed as you relax the tiny muscles around each eye..... 7...........now relax your jaw...................6.......... you can even relax your tongue just by thinking about it......5......soften and relax the back of your neck......4......... and allow that feeling of relaxation to travel down to the shoulders……. Just letting them go…………3…….. and relaxing your upper back…………2…….now your spine……………. all the way down………………1 ……..and finally release the entire body……….0 …..

As you continue to relax I want you to imagine that your conscious mind now sleeps…… and your unconscious mind…..your powerful unconscious mind… wakes……. Opening up almost like a flower……. Unfolding….. Rising and becoming open to all of the wonderful suggestions that I am about to offer …….

//

And as you allow your unconscious mind to slowly awaken……allow the deep inner knowing to pay attention also…… this is the part of you that knows everything about you… your powerful unconscious mind… is the part of you… that can easily, quickly and naturally reprogram your habits and that is why as I speak to you today…… it is so important…. So very important that you allow your unconscious to open up and blossom … to become open… open to the ideas… and just open to the wonderful suggestions that you're going to receive during this session… wonderful ideas… and positive suggestions that will give you that focus… that will give you that discipline… that will give you that motivation to choose a positive action, over an unhealthy action… wonderful ideas and positive suggestions that will bring into your life so many good things… that will bring into your life so many positive things…

As you relax more… your unconscious mind… your powerful unconscious mind… powerfully and completely accepts the idea… that you are now ready to experience extreme weight loss… your subconscious mind powerfully and completely accepts the suggestion that you are ready to choose an alternative to addictive foods… and every time the idea floats into your mind or pops up on a TV screen… this wonderful idea… this positive suggestion… this belief that you are finally ready for extreme weight loss is growing, and getting deeper, and causing you to feel excited, and happy and extremely positive….. this wonderful idea… it grows strong for you… it grows powerful for you… and that's not because I say so… it's because this is the idea… this is the suggestion that you want in your life… and because it's the idea… and because it's the suggestion that you do want in your life… it means… it does simply mean this wonderful idea… it does simply mean this wonderful belief… This positive suggestion grows strong for you… and it grows powerful for you…overriding and overtaking all other ideas and beliefs in your mind that relate to weight loss and your relationship with food…

//

You see now that you are deeply relaxed and your subconscious mind is present here with me now….I want to speak to you honestly and candidly about your addiction to food…. As with all addictions the need to soothe your pain and heal your wound would have led you to indulge in sugary, processed foods that are designed to hook you… the cheap processed foods designed to give you a high…. To make you forget your worries for a moment…. And I want you to know that you are not to blame for becoming addicted to food… this is a common addiction and you so you are not alone…. I also need you to know that you can overcome this addiction…. Despite food being everywhere and easily accessible…. You can learn to soothe your pain in other ways…. In an appropriate way…. In effective ways… in ways that will help you to experience extreme weight loss …..

///

I want you to know that I understand why you made the choice to eat your pain…. To stuff those emotions down and as a result you developed an addiction….I know it wasn't intentional when you first binged on cookies as a small child……this would have worked for you as a small child…. Or even as a teenager….I know you agree that this was a great easy way to soothe all of your pain…. You did what you could to help yourself…. To protect yourself…… to cover those wounds…… but they are still there…. In fact those wounds…. Those same wounds have now become another wound…. They have become the wounds of self doubt…… of low confidence….. of self hatred…… of despair and disappointment in yourself…… all because your comfort has become a burden….. That's right the one thing that seemed to help is now harming you……. That's right stuffing your feelings with food has caused you to become overweight….. Unhealthy addictive foods have caused you to become sad and depressed about your body and caused you to hate the way you look…..andI want you to know that food is not your saviour…. In fact food is simply fuel for your body….. It isn't the cure for your pain and suffering….. it is the fuel for you to move… to think… to live a happy life…. And I know that you are ready to let go of overeating…. to let go of your addiction to food…. And I know you are desperately seeking extreme weight loss…….. And the positive life affirming habits that will help you to heal those wounds and become happy…. Healthy….. Fun and free….

And I want you to know that I am here to help you to release the need to eat when you feel sad or unhappy… I want you to know that you can choose another way and as a result of these new choices accept that….now that you are completely ready for extreme weight loss…..

You are ready to track your weight daily…. You are ready to choose every mouthful you eat carefully….and when you eat… just eat…. To focus on your meal…..and not be doing anything else …… because you know now that the brain can only focus on one thing at a time …… and because you know this you are willing to focus on each and every mouthful savouring the taste…. the smell… the texture and the subtleties of the flavour and sensations of the food you are eating…… you want to make sure you notice the signals from your body about whether or not the food actually agrees with you …… you want to be present to the signal that lets you know this food is good and nutritious…… you want to be in tune with your body and notice how much of the food you are eating you need…..

///

You know now and your unconscious mind is willing to accept the suggestion that you'll enjoy your food more but end up eating less because you're satisfied sooner….. And your unconscious mind is also willing to accept that the more you taste, the less you need….. And so you will eat in only a mindful fashion… you will choose food only when you are truly hungry and you will choose to eat healthy... nutritious foods... in small quantities.... At least every 4 - 6 hours apart..... And your unconscious mind accepts all of this very gratefully now.....

///

The knowledge and understanding your unconscious mind is receiving now means that you are ready to introduce exercise.... Meditation.... and sleep as an alternative to food when you are feeling emotional... stressed or ... even when you want to celebrate..... You will choose a long walk or bike ride as a reward for a good day's work.... You will count your steps daily.... You will stand more and sit less... in fact you are now ready to become a completely different person .... You are ready to become the person that sees sugary food as poison... as an addictive poison that is toxic to your body...... .and it just feels normal and it just feels natural for you to make the right food choices each and every single day... it feels normal and it just feels natural for you to make the right food choices each and every single day because you're in control... you're in complete control of your mind... your body.... Your happiness... and most of all.... You are in control of food.... Food is no longer in control of you......

//

You do find it easy... and because you find it so easy to choose when to eat and what to eat.... it means you're moving now towards a new weight... it means you're moving now towards a size that feels proper and feels completely right for you... and you're moving towards a lower weight... you're moving towards a size that feels proper and feels just right for you because you're now choosing to address your triggers in other ways .. and you're making new choices because you are focused... because you're disciplined... because you feel and you just are motivated... and you have reclaimed control of your life.....

/

...and because you're now willing to accept and let go of your food addiction and addictive foods it means you're becoming... it means you're feeling slimmer... it means you're feeling...
it means you're now becoming healthier... it means you're ready now to accept extreme weight loss into your life...

You are now very deeply relaxed and because you are so relaxed you begin to feel free from all tension, anxiety and fear.......You now realize that you are more confident and sure of yourself because you have taken this enormous step toward helping yourself............ You begin to feel this strength from within, motivating you to overcome any and every obstacle that may stand in the way of your happiness and your freedom from food addiction.

You find that from this moment on you are developing more self-control………… You will now face every situation in a calm, relaxed state of mind. Your thinking is very clear and sharp at all times……….You begin to feel that your self-respect and confidence are expanding more every day in every way.

///

You realize that in the past, overeating, especially sugary processed foods was an escape and food had the control….. Now that you are committed to extreme weight loss, you realize that you must take back the control and reject unhealthy foods…. You are now ready to take full control and carefully choose everything that goes into your mouth…..and by choosing to eat small portions of healthy clean food only when you are hungry it is helping you to become a much happier person with a positive attitude towards life…

You are succeeding in so many areas of your life and you have all the abilities necessary for you to break the overeating pattern………..You choose to be free from food addiction. This is your decision…….You are now doing it…. You are so excited to face your next food challenge…. You can't wait to reject sugary…. Unhealthy food…. Because now you know that you can be and in fact you are back in control of your body….. Whatever happens…. Whenever it happens your first response will be to breathe nice and deeply….you will forget about food…. You will think about walking… running…. Jogging or even dancing….. You will immediately respond to stress with the urge to move your body… you will always choose movement…. you will always choose deep breathing…. You will maintain control over your mind and body….

///

Your desire to be free of food addiction is so important to you that if someone should suggest a dinner…. A buffet or a celebratory slice of cake…. to you, you will find that their reasons for eating are not good enough and that your reasons for rejecting this habit of eating your emotions are far more important…………..

You are always free to make choices and decisions for your own wellbeing and you choose now to be free of food addiction. You know that overeating and indulging in addictive foods is unhealthy and more importantly the cause of your weight gain….overeating brings a lot of unhappiness into your life. At one time you felt that it was a good idea to eat your feelings and stuff them down under a ton of chocolate cake or pizza. It served a purpose in your life at that time. Now… today… with all that you know and have learned during this session…. overeating… turning to food for comfort no longer serves that purpose……….

You realize that addictive foods are a death trap and ultimately, you will never lose weight and keep it off by eating addictive foods…….You are now making a new decision for yourself. You choose the path to real health and happiness. You now choose to be free from food addiction and you are determined to make this happen for you.

You are now proving your inner strength to yourself and to others each and every time that you refuse to indulge................ You know that this is only a bad habit and you can overcome a habit............ So you are choosing to change this particular habit................. You are beginning to find that there are two things which give you more pleasure than addictive foods................ First, you find that you want to take a nice long deep breath whenever you think of eating dirty foods............... This nice long deep breath will help you to feel more calm, more relaxed, and you will feel very peaceful inside. Your mind and body will become calm and relaxed, too calm and relaxed to need to indulge in any type of unhealthy foods.........

You will decide to put off eating dirty foods until some time in the future and when that time comes you forget about them................ Taking a nice long deep breath makes you feel so good, so calm and so relaxed that you will no longer have any desire to eat sugary or processed foods................... Rather you will put it off to some time in the future and you will forget to seek out or eat any addictive foods at that time................. You now find that you are getting hungry at mealtimes and you find a great deal of enjoyment in the healthy and nourishing foods that you eat.......... You find that you want to eat only good nutritious food and as you eat you satisfy any cravings with fruit, vegetables and small portions of good healthy nourishing food instead of with addictive foods...........

///

As of now, you have a very strong unbreakable determination to be free from the addiction to food. With each passing day, your determination to be free becomes stronger and stronger..........until eventually it is no longer a consideration... in fact you look forward to the day when you completely forget that you ever had an addiction to food... and that day is closer than you think... in fact that day will come so quickly.... That being addicted to food will be a distant memory sooner than you think.... And Imagine how that would feel.... Knowing that you once had a food addiction ....so long ago that nobody would ever believe it.....

As soon as this session is over you will awaken with a strong urge that will grow with each passing day to avoid overeating and unhealthy foods.... ....With each passing day and with each moment that goes by you realize that your desire and your self-determination to be free of food addiction is stronger than the hold that food used to have on you. ....

You know now that the answer to extreme weight loss is very simple.... Reject unhealthy foods and eat for nutrition and fuel...... you are already free of food addiction.... And once you return to your daily life you will notice that for short periods of time you will reject dirty foods.....and as each hour passes as each day goes by.... Your need to stay away from dirty foods increases..... for longer and longer periods of time ....and you are eating less dirty, sugary foods.............

You have great confidence in yourself that you can, in fact, be free of dirty addictive foods and that you can do it. Whenever you avoid eating dirty addictive foods in situations where you would have eaten them before, you feel very, very proud of yourself and very sure that you did the right thing for yourself..........

You are now so determined to regain your health and get back to your normal weight, the weight that you should be, that you now gain complete control over your habit. Control means that you not only have the power to walk away from sugar, but that, in fact, you do just that................ You can do it. And each time you do walk away from dirty food.... you find it easier to walk away from the next temptation. You are getting stronger and stronger and very proud of your new strength to walk away from dirty food ....

You are now getting the help you need and you are proud of yourself for having reduced your addictive food habit. You feel good...... And you know, it's so easy to forget something that is no longer important to you.......... We are forgetting all the time - just like you'd probably forgotten about the shoes on your feet until this moment when I mentioned them, and just like you'd probably forgotten what you had for dinner yesterday - we all forget what is no longer important to remember.

And you can forget to eat sugary or processed foods and remember what it's like to feel really good.............. Remember the good feelings now, because you are in control of your life - that's right, you're in complete control of your mind, your body and your health...........

And every day you're feeling better and healthier and fitter and happier. For the first time in ages, you begin to feel really alive. Alive and vibrant, each day is special to you, each day is important to you, each day you become more and more in control of your wonderful life...........And even when things aren't running as smoothly as you'd like, you feel good, because you accept the rough with the smooth, which makes you feel even more in control, even more, certain of your abilities to remain in control, of your life, your mind and your body.

So I'm going to be quiet for a moment or two, to allow you to reflect on these wonderful changes that are occurring within you, right now - that's right, they're occurring deep down at a cellular level, at the very centre of your being.

That's wonderful. Now in a moment, I am going to count from 0 - 5 and on 5 you will open your eyes and it will be as if you were never in a hypnotic state... and you will be ready to move forward and adopt a new way of eating every day...

And 1... ... 2... 3 ...4.....5......and eyes open and welcome back!

Thank you for listening to this powerful hypnotic experience, brought to you by_____

Remember, the results will continue to develop long after this session has finished. And each time you listen, the results get progressively deeper.

Session 4: Extreme Weight Loss No More Emotional Eating

Overview: This session will address the patterns of emotional eating that is a deep-rooted response to the stressors of life, most likely created during childhood. The listener will experience a relaxing induction, deep deepener, allowing them to reset their emotional responses to a healthy alternative, in place of eating.

Time: 30-minutes

[Reader Notes]

- Read the following script at a steady pace, taking your time to guide the listener with your voice.
- Allow long comfortable pauses in between passages, that you are happy with, and follow the key set out below to allow longer pauses.

[Pause Key]

/ Short pause: Reader pauses for 10 seconds

// Medium pause: Reader pauses for 20 seconds

/// Long pause: Reader pauses for 30 seconds

[Script begins]

Hello and welcome to session 4 in the Extreme Weight Loss Series where we will be addressing emotional eating.

At least 30 % of the food many of us eat is non-hungry eating. It is so easy to find yourself eating because you're sad, angry, bored, lonely, stressed, depressed, procrastinating, celebrating, or even commiserating…. the list is endless. Eating for emotions is an extremely common behaviour that is prevalent in today's society. The trouble with eating when you're not hungry is that your body doesn't need the energy and so will take those extra calories and store it as body fat.

This hypnosis audio will reprogram your mind, overriding the habit of emotional eating and replacing it with the mental ability to process your emotions in a healthy manner. My name is _____ and I'll be your guide during this experience.

Take a long deep breath, fill up your lungs and when you exhale, close your eyes …. let yourself relax…..Now put your awareness on your eyelids…. And relax those eyes so deeply……….And when you know that you've done that, hold on to that relaxation.

//

Notice how good it feels. That quality of relaxation you are allowing in your eyes is the quality of relaxation I'd like you to let yourself have throughout your entire body. So take that same quality, bring it up to the top of your head...

/

And I'd like you to focus completely on my voice.... Regardless of any cravings, any uncertain emotions or any desire to eat that may be present now..... And the more you focus on my voice and the words that I say to you..... The faster these thoughts of food and cravings will pass......

/

And back to the relaxation....send it down through your body from the top of your head to the tip of your toes.

Let go of every muscle. Let go of every nerve. Let go of every fibre... And let yourself drift much, deeper, relaxing.....

Now let's really deepen this state.

///

Sit back, breathe deeply, and send a warm feeling into your toes and feet. Let this feeling break up any strain or tension, and as you exhale let the tension drain away. Breathe deeply and send this warm feeling into your ankles. It will break up any strain or tension, and as you exhale let the tension drain away. Breathe deeply and send this feeling into your knees, let it break up any strain or tension there, and as you exhale let the tension drain away. Send this warm sensation into your thighs so any strain or tension is draining away. Breathe deeply and send this warm feeling into your genitals and drain away any tension.

///

Send this warm feeling into your abdomen now; all your internal organs are soothed and relaxed and any strain or tension is draining away. Let this energy flow into your chest and breasts; let it soothe you and as you exhale any tension is draining away. Send this energy into your back now. This feeling is breaking up any strain or tension and as you exhale the tension is draining away. The deep, relaxing energy is flowing through your back, into each vertebra, as each vertebra assumes its proper alignment. The healing energy is flowing into all your muscles and tendons, and you are relaxed, very fully relaxed. Send this energy into your shoulders and neck; this energy is breaking up any strain or tension and as you exhale the tension is draining away. Your shoulders and neck are fully relaxed. And the deep relaxing energy is flowing into your arms; your upper arms, your elbows, your forearms, your wrists, your hands, your fingers are fully relaxed.

Let this relaxing energy wash up over your throat, and your lips, your jaw, your cheeks are fully relaxed. Send this energy into your face, the muscles around your eyes, your forehead, your scalp are relaxed. Any strain or tension is draining away. You are relaxed, almost completely relaxed.

As you relax more and more with each breath... your unconscious... your powerful unconscious mind... the part of you... the part of your mind that knows everything about you... the part of your mind that can easily and naturally help you to be disciplined...

//

your unconscious mind does now begin to become open... open to the suggestions... open
to the wonderful ideas that you're going to receive today... wonderful suggestions... and wonderful ideas that will help you to be absolutely free... free from emotional eating.... Free from the desire to turn to food as a comfort.... Free from the urge to eat food when you experience intense emotions ... free from the need to soothe with food... and you will become free in a really simple easy way..... You will free yourself right now.... In a matter of minutes with simple self-discipline.... That's right self discipline... older than time... your unconscious mind now fully and now completely accepts the suggestion... the wonderful suggestion... that your self-discipline is growing stronger and stronger with every single passing day... that's right... with every single day that passes by... your self-discipline is growing stronger and stronger... and this wonderful suggestion... this wonderful idea is growing strong in your mind... this wonderful suggestion... this wonderful idea is now becoming your true real reality... and that's not because I say so... but simply because this is the suggestion... this is the idea... and this is the wonderful positive change that you want in your life... and because it's the suggestion... because it's the idea... and because it's the positive change that you want in your life... well that means... that your unconscious mind is fully and is completely accepting the suggestion... the wonderful idea... that your self-discipline is growing stronger and stronger with every single passing day...

///

and as you relax more and more now... I want you now to spend a few moments... spend a few moments now thinking about what you want... spend a few moments thinking about what you want... and I'll give you a few moments to think about what it is you do want...

good... and this image... this vision... it grows bright inside your mind... this wonderful vision... this wonderful image just becomes clearer and clearer... and brighter and brighter... this wonderful vision... this wonderful image just helps you now to feel... it just helps you to be disciplined... it helps you to feel... it just helps you to be absolutely motivated...

and you really are a motivated person... you're disciplined... and because you're disciplined... and because you're motivated... and because your discipline is growing stronger and stronger with every single passing day... this wonderful image... this wonderful vision... is growing stronger and stronger... and it's becoming brighter and brighter for you...

//

And you've now become so deeply relaxed... that your mind has become so sensitive... so receptive to what I say... that everything I put into your mind will sink so deeply into the unconscious part of your mind... and will cause so deep and lasting an impression that nothing will eradicate it... and these things... these wonderful positive suggestions that I put into your unconscious mind... will begin to exercise a greater and greater influence over the way you think... over the way you feel... over the way you behave...

and because these things will remain firmly embedded in the unconscious part of your mind... day by day... week by week... month by month... each and every day you'll discover and you begin to feel... calmer and calmer... more and more relaxed... because from this moment on each and every day... you're going to experience a greater feeling of well-being... physical as well as mental well-being...

/

...and each and every day I would like you just to know... that with each day that goes by you're going to become a little more mentally calm... and more and more clear in your mind... each and every day... which means that you're going to be able to think more clearly... to see things more clearly... so that nothing and no one will ever be able to worry you... or upset you in quite the same way... your mind is becoming more and more clear... crystal clear... allowing you to feel physically more relaxed... more relaxed in your body... more relaxed about yourself... more relaxed about the world around you...

/

and as the days... and the weeks... and the months go by... and you become ever more calm... ever more clear in your mind... ever more relaxed in your body... it will be perfectly natural that you're going to be able to cope better... with anything and anybody... and any situation that you have to handle in your daily life... because you're coping more calmly... more and more confidently, too... more confidently... because you have greater self-control... greater control over the way you think... greater control over the way you feel... and greater control over the way you do things... and the way you behave...

each and every day... you're going to experience a greater feeling of well-being... physical as well as mental well-being... and a greater feeling of safety and security to... than you've experienced in a long... long time... and all together, each and every day... it will feel like a weight... it will feel like a burden is being lifted off your shoulders... allowing you to live your life in a way that's much more satisfying... satisfying to you... and with each and every day that passes by... those things that may have annoyed you... those things that may have caused you unnecessary stresses in your life... those things now no longer seem to affect you in quite the same way... it's almost like those things just wash off you... just like water washes off of a duck's back...

/

and as you continue now to relax more and more with every breath... as you now continue to become more and more calm... more and more relaxed... each and every one of these wonderful positive suggestions... grow stronger and stronger for you... as you continue to relax more and more with every breath... each and every one of these positive suggestions become more and more real for you... so continue now to relax more and more... continue to relax more and more...

and each and every day now... your resolve becomes stronger... you become steadier... each and every day... your mind feels much calmer... clearer... more composed... and each and every day you become stronger and more disciplined... and it becomes a natural way of being for you.... And each day you develop more resolve... you develop more discipline until there is no other way for you to live ....

/

you just find that it becomes much easier for you... and more and more natural for you... to do those things which you know inside your own mind... move you towards your ideal weight... and each and every day as you begin to feel calmer... more and more relaxed... it's beginning to just feel more natural... easier and easier to avoid those foods... those excuses... that you know inside your own mind move you further away from your ideal weight... each and every day you truly are feeling much calmer... more relaxed in yourself...

those things that may have troubled you in the past... those things that used to annoy you... those things that in the past may have made you turn to food... those things now no longer seem to affect you in quite the same way... you truly are, each and every day... just feeling much calmer in yourself... more relaxed... even happier and happier...

because each and every day that passes by now... you truly are doing more and more of those things which you know inside your own mind move you towards your ideal weight... and each and every day... a wonderful belief... a wonderful belief that you can and will reach your ideal weight only grows stronger and stronger for you...

//

and once you've reached your ideal weight... which you will achieve... you'll maintain this belief... you'll stay at the weight that you want to be... and each and every day... these wonderful suggestions grow stronger and stronger for you...

And in a few moments, I am going to bring this session to a close...and when I do you will awaken with a whole new perspective on food, eating and emotions...

And I am going to count from 0 - 3 and on 3 you will open your eyes and it will be as if you were never in a hypnotic state... and you will remember every important lesson that you heard...
And 1... ... 2... 3 and eyes open and welcome back!

Thank you for listening to this powerful hypnotic experience...remember, the results will continue to develop long after this session has finished.... and each time you listen, the results get progressively deeper.

Session 5: Extreme Weight loss Burn Fat Rapidly

Overview: This session will program the mind to seek ways to burn fat rapidly, daily. With a deep relaxation induction and deepener, the hypnotic suggestions included are designed to reprogram any deep-set beliefs around exercise and fat-burning activity.

Time: 30-minutes

[Reader Notes]

- Read the following script at a steady pace, taking your time to guide the listener with your voice.
- Allow long comfortable pauses in between passages, that you are happy with, and follow the key set out below to allow longer pauses.

[Pause Key]

/ Short pause: Reader pauses for 10 seconds

// Medium pause: Reader pauses for 20 seconds

/// Long pause: Reader pauses for 30 seconds

Hello and welcome to this powerful hypnotic session, from _____

[Script Begins]

Hello and welcome to session 5 in the Extreme Weight Loss Series. This powerful hypnotic session is designed to help you to burn fat rapidly through a daily fitness and activity mindset that will develop over the coming days and weeks. All you have to do is relax and focus on my voice. My name is _____ and I'll be your guide during this experience.

There is nothing for you to do except listen to my voice as I guide you into a deep state of relaxation where your conscious mind sleeps and your unconscious mind takes over... and all you need to do to achieve this is breathe.... Nice and deeply...

And just notice how your body moves as you breathe nice and deeply... allowing each breath to fill the entire body... calming the mind and releasing any tightness or tension that may be present in the body... as you contemplate what it will take to burn fat rapidly by achieving the mindset of daily fitness

Close your eyes and begin to relax ... Relax all the muscles in your body and allow yourself to sink deep into the chair ... Take in a deep breath ... and hold it ... wait three seconds. Let it out slowly ... good. Take in another deep breath ... and hold it ... wait three seconds. Let it out slowly ... yes. With each exhale, you will fall deeper and deeper into a more relaxed state of mind ... Take one more deep breath ... and hold it ... wait three seconds. Let it out slowly ... excellent.

//

You are now cleansing your body of all its negative energy. You are cleansing your entire body starting at your feet and ending with the top of your head ... Feel all the muscles in your toes, feet, and ankles ... Visualize the tense and negative energy in your feet as a dark, thick cloud ... Take a deep breath in. Hold. On your exhale, feel this cloud travel up through your body and release with your breath ... Exhale ... Perfect ... Feel all the muscles in your calves, shins, and knees ... Visualize the tense and negative energy in your calves, shins, and knees as a dark, thick cloud ... Take a deep breath in. Hold. On your exhale, feel this cloud travel up through your body

Release with your breath ... Exhale ... Nice ... Feel all the muscles in your pelvis and stomach
... Visualize the tense and negative energy in your pelvis and stomach as a dark, thick cloud ... Take a deep breath in. Hold. On your exhale, feel this cloud travel up through your body and release with your breath... Exhale... ... Feel all the muscles in your chest and back... Visualize the tense and negative energy in your chest and back as a dark, thick cloud ... Take a deep breath in. Hold. On your exhale, feel this cloud travel up through your body and release with your breath... Exhale ... Good ... Feel all the muscles in your arms ... Visualize the tense and negative energy in your arms as a dark, thick cloud ... Take a deep breath in. Hold. On your exhale, feel this cloud travel up through your body and release with your breath ... Exhale ... ... Feel all the muscles in your hands and fingers ... Visualize the tense and negative energy in your hands and fingers as a dark, thick cloud ...

Take a deep breath in. Hold. On your exhale, feel this cloud travel up through your body and release with your breath ... Exhale ... Excellent ... Feel all the muscles in your neck and shoulders ... Visualize the tense and negative energy in your neck and shoulders as a dark, thick cloud ... Take a deep breath in. Hold. On your exhale, feel this cloud travel up through your body and release with your breath ... Exhale ... ... Visualize any remaining tense and negative energy in any part of your body as a dark, thick cloud ... Take a deep breath in. Hold.....On your exhale, feel this cloud... travel up through your body and release with your breath ... Exhale ... Perfect ... Your body is now free of all stress. There is nothing you need to do and nowhere you need to be ... Each breath you take cleans your body, mind, and spirit, drifting you deeper and deeper into the depths of your subconscious mind.

//

You are now totally focused on your breathing ... Take in a deep breath ... and hold it... wait three seconds. Let it out slowly ... Take in another deep breath ... and hold it... wait three seconds. Let it out slowly ... with each exhale, you will drift deeper and deeper into a more relaxed state of mind.

And even as you begin to drift deeper into this comfortable state of relaxation, you are aware of the sound of my voice – and the words that you hear during this hypnotic trance will have an immediate and permanent effect on the way that you think and feel.

///

Now that you are feeling more relaxed and comfortable – I want you to visualize you are calmly walking down a peaceful hallway....in front of you, you see the soft lights of beautiful candles flickering on either side of the hallway.......you can smell the sweet scent of the candles...feeling very calm and relaxed as you walk down the hallway...As you walk calmly, you notice there are 10 windows that hold these candles throughout the hall...as you walk past these windows with candles, I want you to visualize the candles slowly flicker out as you pass by...with each flickering candle, you are lead deeper and deeper into relaxation.

The candles will lead you down, down, down...these are the candles that will lead you deep into relaxation...and in a moment, as I begin to count, you will envision yourself calmly walking down this hallway, past the first candle lit window...and then the next....you will find the further down the hallway you walk...flickering out the candles... the more comfortable and relaxed you become.
I am going to count as you begin down this hallway full of ten candlelit windows...imagine how peaceful and relaxing this feels as you go past each window...the candles flicker out...and with each candle, you enter deeper and deeper into relaxation...

10 - Deeply relaxed… 9 - Walking further and further 8 - More and more relaxed 7 Deeper and Deeper
6 -5 More and more and more relaxed 4 - Deeply relaxed, further and further 3 - More and more relaxed

2 - Almost to the last window now, just one more set of candles...and 1 - Deep, deep relaxation ... all the way down... Now that you have reached the last window and are totally relaxed....just allow yourself to let go completely as you go deeper and deeper..... In a moment I'm going to relax you more completely … so let's get the mind relaxed, that's really what we want to do. When your mind's relaxed you really can achieve anything you can think of, within certain restrictions of course. In a moment I'll ask you to slowly begin counting out loud, backwards, starting with the number 100.

After each number, simply say the words, 'deeper relaxed'. After each number double your mental relaxation, let your mind grow twice as calm and still and serene.

Now if you do this, you'll discover by the time you just say a couple of numbers, it doesn't take long, you've relaxed your mind so beautifully and so completely, you've actually relaxed all the rest of the numbers out. Want that... And you can have it quickly.

Slowly begin counting out loud, backwards, starting with the number 100. Saying the words, deeper relaxed… And relax those numbers right out of your mind.

"100 deeper relaxed" That's good. "99 deeper relaxed" That's fine.

"98 deeper relaxed."

Now you can let those numbers grow dim and distant, they're not important.

"97 deeper relaxed."

And when you're ready just push them out.

"96 deeper relaxed."

Now push them on out, just tell them to leave and they will go. Just let them go… And let them be gone.

…Numbers all gone ?

When you are starting ..to notice that.. it is becoming easier …..and easier to get ..what you REALLY desire ..can you BEGIN NOW each day to begin… to notice as you …begin finding yourself ..doing things that you ..really enjoy ..that are a part of …getting what you long for ..and as YOU …are feeling lighter …..and you float …..through everything you do …. can you notice you are noticing … that with a sense.. of happiness….you are seeing …that you are getting what you want…. And as you find yourself….. enjoying doing the things… that are helping you ….in getting what you want…. could it be that every day …..you're tingling with excitement….. as you're noticing what you are …..achieving and will achieve…..as you happily get closer to ….what it is that you long for…. And if you find yourself …….each night before sleeping ……enjoying writing down your fitness or exercise achievements ……for that day ………and making all the wonderful workout plans….. for tomorrow…..could you notice ……that you find yourself getting …..even more excited, ……encouraged and ecstatic… about fitness and exercise …. and noticing what it is ……that you're getting out of life.

And if with every breath ……you are taking you start to ……realize that you are becoming……. more excited about exercise as you …..are realizing that with ……..every breath you are taking ….. you are getting closer to ….what you long for. …..rapid fat burning ….that is ….. And you're seeing ….everything clearly, finally your fitness life is becoming clearer…..you're feeling excited …..and you're so happy…. And you know, you know …..where that power comes from….. as it fills your heart ..and it beats each day… of your life…… with the images of ……your fitness desires and exercise accomplishments…. And you know you know ……what you can do….. to get what you want as you easily achieve ……..your fitness goals and dreams.

And from this moment on you exercise on a regular basis… and exercise is something that you enjoy doing… you exercise on a regular basis… and exercising on a regular basis is something that you enjoy doing… and this wonderful suggestion of exercising on a regular basis and enjoying it… this wonderful suggestion now grows strong for you inside your mind… this wonderful suggestion of exercising on a regular basis and enjoying it… becomes more and more real for you each and every day… and that's not because I say so… it's simply because it's the suggestion that you want working in your life…

…and because it is the suggestion that you want working in your life… it now does mean that you will burn fat rapidly by exercising on a regular basis… and exercising on a regular basis is something that you enjoy… from this moment on… you always find the time to exercise… you always find the time to exercise… you always find the time to exercise… because exercising is important to you… exercise allows you to achieve your goals with ease…

….and because you do exercise on a regular basis… that now means that with each and every day that passes… you feel healthier… you feel fitter… and that's because you always… absolutely always… feel motivated to exercise because exercise makes you feel good… exercise allows you to achieve your goals with ease…. you feel motivated to exercise because you enjoy it…

……and because you do exercise on a regular basis… that does now mean that you're getting the figure that you deserve… and all these wonderful positive suggestions of exercising on a regular basis… enjoying exercise… being motivated and determined to exercise… all these wonderful suggestions now grow strong inside your mind… all of these wonderful suggestions now become more real for you… not because I say so but simply because these are the suggestions that you want working in your life…

and now in a few moments… I'm going to count from one to three… and at the count of three… I want you to imagine yourself in your mind's eye exercising… I want you to imagine yourself exercising… feeling good… enjoying it… and feeling those wonderful positive endorphins filling your entire body… so one… two… three…

imagine yourself now exercising… imagine how good you feel… how much you're enjoying it… and begin to feel those wonderful positive endorphins filling your entire body… imagine that in your mind's eye right now… and I'll give you a few moments to do that…

///

and continue now to relax more and more… continue to relax just more and more, with each breath… relax…more and more… relax… more with each breath…

and in a few moments again I will count from one to three… and this time, at the count of three… I want you to imagine in your mind's eye… imagine yourself looking into a mirror… noticing how much slimmer… healthier… and fitter you look because of the exercise that you've been doing… and then imagine thinking to yourself how good it feels to be like this… so one… two… three…

imagine yourself there looking into a mirror… noticing how slim, healthy and fit you look…. just thinking to yourself how good it feels to be like this… imagine that… and I'll give you a few moments to do that…

///

good… and you can now just feel good knowing that the image will be your true reality… simply because of the fact that you exercise on a regular basis… and in a few moments… I'm going to help you to create that belief… that you exercise on a regular basis and enjoy it… I will help you to create that belief … in a few moments; I'm going to repeat the suggestion… I exercise on a regular basis and I enjoy it…

///

…now when I say that suggestion… all I'd like you to do is to mentally repeat that suggestion to yourself, inside your mind… because each and every time that you do that… each and every time that you mentally repeat that suggestion to yourself… inside your mind… it makes that belief that you exercise on a regular basis and enjoy it more real for you… stronger and stronger… so as I say the suggestion… mentally repeat it to yourself… so let's begin…

I exercise on a regular basis and I enjoy it… and again say to yourself…

I exercise on a regular basis and I enjoy it…

I exercise on a regular basis and I enjoy it…

I exercise on a regular basis and I enjoy it… I exercise on a regular basis and I enjoy it…

and every time that you just mentally repeat that suggestion to yourself… your belief in the suggestion grows stronger and stronger… and becomes more and more real… so again say to yourself…

I exercise on a regular basis and I enjoy it…

I exercise on a regular basis and I enjoy it…

I exercise on a regular basis and I enjoy it… I exercise on a regular basis and I enjoy it… once more, say to yourself…

I exercise on a regular basis and I enjoy it…

and you do exercise on a regular basis… and exercising is something that you enjoy doing… and from this moment on… whenever you say the word…

exercise… to yourself inside your mind… you instantly feel motivated to go and exercise… that's right… from this moment on… every time that you just mentally say to yourself that word…

exercise… you instantly feel motivated to go and exercise…

and each and every time that you use this suggestion… each and every time that you repeat that trigger word…

exercise

you feel more and more motivated to exercise… and each and every time that you listen to this session… the wonderful positive effects grow much stronger for you… each and every time that you listen to this session… the wonderful positive suggestions only become more and more real for you…

And in a few moments, I am going to bring this session to a close…and when I do you will awaken excited about the prospect of exercising daily and enjoying your new found fitness status…

And I am going to count from 0 - 5 and on 5 you will open your eyes and it will be as if you were never in a hypnotic state… and you will be ready to exercise and workout every day with ease…..

And 1… … 2… 3 …4…..5……and eyes open and welcome back!

Thank you for listening to this powerful hypnotic experience….remember, the results will continue to develop long after this session has finished. And each time you listen, the results get progressively deeper.

Bonus Session:
Extreme Weight Loss Affirmations

Overview: This affirmation session is designed to reprogram any negative self-talk that the
The listener has developed over years of unhealthy eating habits, emotional eating and food addiction.

Time: 30-minutes *[Repeat the affirmations 3 times for them to take effect in the mind of the listener.]*

[Reader Notes]

- Read the following script at a steady pace, taking your time to guide the listener with your voice.
- Allow long comfortable pauses in between passages, that you are happy with, and follow the key set out below to allow longer pauses.

Hello and welcome to this powerful hypnotic session, from _____ *[Script Begins]*

Hello and welcome to this powerful affirmation session…..

As we discussed in an earlier session, self-talk is one of the secrets to developing an Extreme Weight Loss mindset, and in this session you will add a series of powerful messages to your self-talk vocabulary, making it effortless for you to tell yourself the things that will add to your Extreme Weight Loss.

These Extreme Weight Loss Affirmations are extremely powerful and can be listened to while working, commuting, or sleeping. Listen to this audio daily for a minimum of 40 days for best results.

Relax, and enjoy!

Every day in every way I am getting smaller and smaller

Every day in Every way I biome more open to the idea of Extreme Weight Loss

Every day in every way I am getting fitter and fitter

Extreme Weight Loss is now a part of my life

Losing weight finally is a part of who I am

When I gain weight, losing those extra pounds will be a natural response for me.

I am comfortably and happily achieving my weight loss goals.

I am committed to losing weight every day.

I am excited about my new urge to exercise regularly.

I am open to the idea of eating foods that contribute to my health and wellbeing.

I am ready to finally eat only when I am hungry.

I am now clear about my ideal weight.

I am falling in love with the taste of healthy food.

I am gaining more and more control each and every day of how much I eat.

I am creating an Extreme Weight Loss mindset every day

Every day as soon as I open my eyes I have a strong desire to exercise and move my body I am enjoying exercising, it makes me feel really good.

I am becoming fitter and stronger every day through exercise. I am easily

reaching and maintaining my ideal weight I truly love and care for my mind and

body.

I am ready to live a long healthy life and I accept that requires Extreme Weight Loss I am finally ready to accept that I deserve to have a slim, healthy, attractive body.

I am developing more healthy eating habits all the time.

I do what it takes to be healthy.

I have happily redefined weight loss success.

I make the hard decision every day to choose to exercise.

I am developing a real taste for nutritious, real foods

I am committed to eating foods that create a sense of hope and success deep within me I finally accept full responsibility for my weight, my life and my own health.

I have made the decision to fall in love with my body daily.

I finally believe in myself and my ability to succeed.

I have hope and certainty about my new weight loss future.

I finally accept fully, that it is time for me to change my body

I have decided that I am ready to enjoy everything that nourishes and strengthens my body and mind.

I finally understand that making small changes makes the difference in extreme weight loss.

I recognise how much I enjoy the feeling of well-being these changes are giving me.

I love myself and as a result, I accept all of my previous mistakes and learn from them. I accept the past for what it is and rather than looking back I will change my weight for the future.

I am committed to saying no to addictive food when I need to.

I exercise to enjoy a strong, toned body.

I am falling in love with the feeling that exercise gives me.

It does not matter what other people say or do.

I am confident in my ability to choose to believe in myself.

Today I choose to manage my emotions with meditation and mindfulness

I am ready to choose to surround myself with healthy, slim, people who also manage their weight.

I look forward to achieving my ideal weight.

I am patient with creating my better body.

I am committing myself to my weight loss journey

I am happy with every small or large thing I do in my great effort to lose weight.

Every day I am becoming smaller and healthier.

I accept that I am in the process of developing an attractive body.

I am creating a body that I like and enjoy.

I accept that changing my eating habits is the crux of changing my body I celebrate my own inner power to make good choices around food.

I am loving my new daily walking routine

I am willing to change

I am willing to create new thoughts about myself and my body.

I am willing to work hard on my Extreme Weight Loss journey

I am excited about my future as a result of my Extreme Weight Loss journey

I am delighted about my new ideal size and weight

I choose to embrace thoughts of confidence in my ability to make positive changes in my life.

It feels good to move my body.

I accept that exercise can be fun!

I use deep breathing to help me relax and handle stress. I am worthy of a

healthy, smaller, fitter body I deserve to be at my ideal weight.

Now I have the tools, it is finally safe for me to lose weight.

I release all judgment around my previous struggles and embrace my Extreme Weight Loss journey

I actually have a powerful metabolism I maintain my body with optimal health.

I accept my body shape and acknowledge the ideal weight for me I let go of unhelpful patterns of behaviour around food.

I embrace even the most difficult choices and decisions for my higher good.

I let go of any guilt I hold around food choices.

I am grateful for the body I own and all it does for me.

I am active and full of energy.

I am developing a craving for healthy nutritious foods daily. I breathe through any sugar or processed food cravings Today I choose to heal and nourish my body.

I value self-control and self-mastery of my eating habits and daily movement

I recognize what has not been working for me in the past, and I have the courage to change.

I've conquered my impulsive nature, and choose food with intention and integrity.

I wake up each day with a clear determination to reach my ideal weight.

Each time I resist temptation, I strengthen my own self-mastery.

I eat well, sleep well, and exercise well.

I enjoy every bite when I eat.

I enjoy taking a moment to think before I eat.

Every cell in my body gets regenerated by a good night's sleep I enjoy moving my body and feeling my heart pumping.

I am free of food addiction

I am now a fan of vegetables, fruits and whole foods.

My metabolism is running optimally, helping me achieve my desired weight.

I let go of the guilt I have around food.

I breathe in relaxation and breathe out stress.

My journey is unique and I do not compare myself to other people who are also losing weight.

My food choices are consistent with my desire to be my optimal weight.

I am on a lifelong path of wellness.

Each day I recommit to my journey of Extreme Weight Loss

Extreme Weight Loss Hypnosis: Guided Meditations, Affirmations& Self-Hypnosis For Food Addiction, Emotional Eating, Rapid Fat Burning, Mindfulness & Healthy Deep Sleep Habits

By

Jessica Jacobs

© Copyright 2021 - All rights reserved.

The content contained within this book may not be reproduced, duplicated or transmitted without direct written permission from the author or the publisher.

Under no circumstances will any blame or legal responsibility be held against the publisher, or author, for any damages, reparation, or monetary loss due to the information contained within this book; either directly or indirectly.

Legal Notice:

This book is copyright protected. This book is only for personal use. You cannot amend, distribute, sell, use, quote or paraphrase any part, or the content within this book, without the consent of the author or publisher.

Disclaimer Notice:

Please note the information contained within this document is for educational and entertainment purposes only. All effort has been executed to present accurate, up to date, and reliable, complete information. No warranties of any kind are declared or implied. Readers acknowledge that the author is not engaging in the rendering of legal, financial, medical or professional advice.

Table of Contents

Introduction 53

Induction 54

Deepening 56

Reduce the Portions Size 59

Get Rid of the Sweet Tooth 61

Low Carbohydrate Diet 64

Self-Hypnosis 67

Protective Sleep 70

Relaxing Sleep 74

Be Healthy 77

Be More Active 78

Maintenance Insomnia Relaxation 79

Inner Strength and Power 81

Connect with Your Special Place 84

Have a strong belief in yourself 85

Affirmations 87

To the Narrator

Introduction - 5 min long

Induction – Beach 20 min long

Deepener – Beach 20 min long

Get rid of the Mind Clutter 15 min long

Reduce the Portions Size 20 min long

Get Rid of the Sweet Tooth 15 min long

Low Carbohydrate Diet 15 min long

Self-Hypnosis 12 min long

Protective Sleep 15 min long

Relaxing Sleep 20 min long

Be Healthy 15 min long

Be More Active 10 min long

Maintain Insomnia Relaxation 20 min long

Inner Strength and Power 20 min long

Connect with Your Special Space 5 min long
Have a Strong belief in Yourself 15 min long

Affirmations 60 min long

"…" means take a breath while speaking before you continue.

PAUSE (for a few breaths)

LONGER PAUSE (give time to allow the listener time to imagine what you've suggested)

Introduction

Thank you for listening to Extreme Weight Loss Hypnosis: Guided Meditations, Affirmations& Self-Hypnosis For Food Addiction, Emotional Eating, Rapid Fat Burning, Mindfulness & Healthy Deep Sleep Habits audio

… this surely is a sign of awareness and self-love. This only means that you want to burn fat, lose weight with the help of hypnosis and mindfulness …to be able to feel and look great.

Pause

So, congratulations for taking this step towards a fitter and happier YOU…please listen to this audio using headphones… so that the sound of my voice is clear and if you lose track of me and your mind starts to wander…you can easily tune back into the sound of my voice.

Pause

Do not listen to this audio…when your mind needs you to be conscious such as while operating machinery or driving. Listen to this audio… when you are in a comfortable position…sitting on a chair or resting on a bed.

Pause

Induction

Take a deep breath in and gently close your eyes. Draw your attention to your body and start to relax. Let your next inhale be long and deep… Filling your lungs to the brim… And then gently releasing with a slow exhale through your mouth…

Pause

You feel twice as relaxed and at ease. With each cycle of breath becoming deeper and longer, you can feel a heavy sense of relaxation settling into every part of your body… Take a deep cleansing breath in, and let a deep relaxing breath out.

Pause

The creative part of your mind begins to take you to a place which will help you relax even further… You will feel more at ease than you have ever before. And now you find yourself standing at a beach, with all five senses soaking in the surroundings.

Pause

As you look around this white sandy beach, you notice that it goes on as far as the eye can see on your left and right. As you turn your gaze to the water, you see the bright clear blues up until the horizon, full of gentle waves. As you look up at the sky, you notice the seagulls flying cheerfully above you, gliding with the pleasantly warm breeze… You now begin walking towards the water, feeling the soft sand beneath your feet…

Pause

Hearing the waves kissing the shore and the seagulls' call. The more you notice these sights and sounds, the more relaxed you become.

As you take a deep relaxing breath in, you can smell the salty seas which relax you even further. You feel deeply at ease and comfortable here. While you are walking towards the shore, you notice some shells in the beach sand… You decide to pause and pick one up. As you draw your attention towards this shell, you can see the light pink and white colours on it…

Pause

You feel the texture of this shell… It feels soft and smooth on one side, and slightly bumpy on the other… You try to place it near your ear and you can hear the melody of the sea waves echoing in it. This puts you more at ease. You place the shell back in the sand and continue walking till you reach a large and cozy blanket... You decide to lie down on it.

Pause

The moment your back touches this cosy blanket, you feel twice as relaxed. The breeze kissing your skin gently as it flows by. You begin to relax your body, starting with your head... Relax the muscles of your forehead and temples... Notice how great that feels. You now bring relaxation to your jaw... Allowing all tension in the muscles to fade away.

Gently move your neck from side to side, allowing the muscles here to relax even further. Carry this relaxation through to the rest of your body, moving now into your chest, shoulders, and arms, all the way to your fingertips... Notice how amazing it feels to be this relaxed. Let this deep relaxation now move into your stomach and back, completely relaxing your upper body before moving to your waist, hips and thighs... Deeply relaxing every muscle here. The further down you go the more relaxed you feel.

Pause

Notice the relaxation flowing into your knees, calves, and shins... Your legs are so relaxed they almost feel limp as this relaxation settles into the soles of your feet and toes. Your entire body is now so deeply relaxed that you feel entirely at ease. Notice the warmth of the breeze and the comfort of the blanket. Soak it all in and enjoy feeling deeply relaxed in the mind and body, as you continue to lay on this blanket.

Deepening

You now begin to gently sit up, and slowly open your eyes to the stunning views of the beach and the sea. As you look out into the horizon, you notice the setting sun lighting up the sky in all shades of crimson, yellow, and purple.

As I now count from 10, you will notice the sun moving closer and closing to the horizon, relaxing you deeply with each count…

Ten, the sun begins to go down slowly…

Nine, the sun moves further down and you feel more and more relaxed…

Eight, you find yourself going deeper into relaxation as the sun gets closer to the horizon…

Seven, the sun is now in touch with the horizon and you're settling into deep relaxation…

Six, the sun is moving further below the horizon and you are settling into hypnosis…

Five, feeling more and more relaxed…

Four, half the sun has set below the horizon and you are moving deeper into relaxation…

Three, drifting deeper still…

Two, the sun has almost disappeared beneath the horizon and at the next number you will be completely and deeply relaxed…

One, you are deeply relaxed, feeling comfortable. We will now focus on bringing helpful changes to your subconscious mind as we go forward.

Get Rid of the Mind Clutter

Begin to slowly but steadily settle into this tranquil state of hypnosis. Here, I would like you to think of a reason that has made you listen to me right now. The problem that you wish to address today is something a lot of people experience every now and then. And in the next few moments I will help walk you through some strategies that will enable you to free yourself from the clutter inside your mind.

Pause

While it is natural for the mind to get cluttered from time to time, it can get bothersome when it occurs while you are trying to fall asleep. However, you must note that the brain never really falls asleep, it is just the body that resorts to rest. And it is when you sleep that the mind begins to sift and sort through the various files it has accumulated through your experiences when you were awake and conscious.

Pause

As your mind begins the task of processing all the information before it, you may at times find it difficult to rest because the speed with which your mind goes through one information to another is just too much. Consequently, it makes your body feel like it cannot relax.

At this moment here, I would like you to picture yourself seated in a cinema hall by yourself. You're sitting at the very back row, far away from the big white screen. The hall is dark and you can see the light from the projector lighting up the screen, shining on it like a beam of light from a lighthouse in the middle of the sea helping you spot the dangers around you.

Pause

The screen on the other hand, is representative of your mind. And as you sit here gazing at the screen, you begin to notice how it fills up with a lot of random things -- both words and images. Even the sound coming from the speakers seems random and difficult to understand.

This is exactly how the clutter inside your mind feels. To put a stop to this is our aim for today.

So, take a deep breath in through your nose, allow your lungs to fill up completely, and then gently exhale through your mouth to relax yourself as you sit here in the cinema hall watching and listening to this clutter.

Pause

With the power of your imagination, I would like you to notice how the random images and words on the screen begin to merge -- coming together and expanding into a huge ball full of all sorts of colours, as if someone was filling air into a ball or a hot air balloon. As all of this unfolds on the big screen, you know how far away from it all you sit, and from this far away it just seems like any other ball or balloon swirling around.

From this far away, you feel relaxed and calm as you watch all the clutter being sucked into the structure of a ball or a balloon. All of the randomness and all the indistinct sounds are getting sucked into this structure little by little.

Pause

Take one more deep breath in through your nose, slowly, noticing your chest expanding with your inhale, and then gently let it all out with an exhale through your mouth. Continue this rhythm of deep breathing and you will notice how the ball or balloon on the screen slowly begins to deflate, becoming smaller and smaller each time you exhale.

By now the ball or balloon on the screen has become so small that you can hardly see it. With a little effort you might spot a small dot somewhere on this giant white screen of your mind.

And now the screen looks completely white as all the clutter in your mind has disappeared. It is now time for you to stand up from your seat in this hall and begin to walk towards the screen in order to incorporate it, complete with all this clarity, back into your mind where it truly belongs.

Pause

Take one step, and then another, and then another, steadily making your way down the aisle beginning to incorporate the screen into your mind with every step you take. And as it begins to settle back into your mind, you feel free from all the clutter.

All of these suggestions that I have spoken, will stay with you and grow stronger and stronger with each passing hour and with each passing day.

Remember, if at any moment in the future you feel the need to clear the clutter in your mind, simply close your eyes, take a deep breath in and as you breathe out, find yourself back in that cinema hall. Doing so will help you once again step away from your thoughts until they diminish and fade away completely, leaving your mind absolutely clear once again.

Pause

Reduce the Portions Size

Having a proper diet and regular exercise plays a pivotal role in boosting the metabolism.

To achieve a high metabolic state, you need to split your meals into smaller portions of 5-6 meals a day, and add in 30 mins of exercise to your daily routine.

This will not only boost your metabolism, but will also help improve your digestion, stabilise your blood sugar levels, and help you feel energised by as your body receives optimum nutrition throughout the day.

By eating smaller portions, you reduce the time gap between meals, and thereby avoid feeling extremely hungry which in turn prevents you from binge eating.

Pause

It is important to eat healthy meals and snacks such as fruits and salads to ensure your body receives all the right nutrients while also making sure you feel satisfied.

And with this change, you will soon notice how all your body parts and organs feel rejuvenated, and you will notice yourself functioning at an optimum level.

With each passing day, you see your energy levels increasing, and you will notice how your metabolism slowly aligns with your bodily needs.

Your conscious and subconscious efforts to reduce the size of your meal portions, and to eat healthy, nutritious food is beneficial for your overall health.

Now, I want you to carefully listen to each and every word I say, and observe yourself slowly beginning to feel calm and relaxed.

You feel a sense of peace and calm within you, and because of all the improvements taking place inside your mind, your body will feel at rest, and your metabolism will readjust.

You pump more air to your lungs, and your heartbeat will become steadier, and your breathing will become natural.

What this means is your nervous system is beginning to function more appropriately, and all your organs are working harmoniously inside your body.

Pause

Now, as you continue to eat only when you are hungry, you will begin to gain confidence, and you will recognize the emotional triggers which drive you to binge eating.

You take charge of your life and your body, and you will no longer eat junk food or comfort food.

And with each passing day, you will gain more control over your eating habits and exercise routine.

You will become more and more focused and you will channel all your energies into effectively accomplishing your goals.

Pause

Now, picture yourself as an attractive, healthy, and confident woman and observe how your goals slowly begin to manifest into reality.

By applying a simple method of paying attention to the portions of your meals, and by slowly becoming more and more aware of your emotional triggers, you begin to eat healthy, avoid junk foods and binge eating, and thereby allowing yourself to feel confident and healthy.

Pause

Isn't it amazing how you already feel so good just by making this crucial decision?

And whenever you feel the need, this recording will help you feel relaxed about achieving your goal of a healthier, attractive and slimmer body.

Get Rid of the Sweet Tooth

I want you to now bring your focus to the sound of my voice, and allow yourself to go into a deeper state of relaxation with every breath you take.

Observe how my words sink deeper into your subconscious mind as you begin to feel more and more comfortable, and relaxed.

You are now aware that desserts, sweetened drinks, and other sugary foods make it harder for you to lose weight. Isn't it? Yes, it is…

Pause

Now pay close attention to my words as it is going to help you eliminate your cravings for sweet and sugary substances.

Pause

Before we go ahead, we are going to take a deeper look into your mind and identify the emotional triggers that make you crave for sugary substances.

Longer Pause

And, now that you have identified these triggers, the time has come to understand the purpose of it.

You are also now aware that you can satisfy these cravings with natural sugars available in fruits, which means you can satiate these cravings without having a negative effect on your body, mind and your goals of a healthier lifestyle.

You are excited about achieving your weight loss goals because you love yourself.

You will now consciously make a deal with your sweet tooth to satiate all it's cravings for sugary substances only from fresh fruits and vegetables.

You are now aware that you can easily substitute sugar with raw honey or jaggery, and this will satiate your sweet tooth which is a win-win situation for you and your sweet tooth cravings.

Pause

Sugary foods and artificially sweetened drinks convert sugar into fat that harden the arteries, and also cause your teeth to rotten quickly.

It is therefore imperative for you to limit these cravings, and when necessary, you satiate these cravings with fruits and vegetables.

You are now conditioning yourself into satiating your sweet tooth cravings with healthier, and naturally available sugar in fruits, vegetables and whole grains.

Pause

Now try and go deeper back into time when you first tasted sugary foods.

Perhaps it was when you were much younger.

Longer Pause

Now I want you to let yourself sink deeper into that time when your younger self first started eating sweets, chocolates, candies and other similar sugary substances.

Maybe, it was your parents or uncles and aunties that gave you these sweets to pacify you.

Whatever the case may be, it's now time for your adult self to go deeper and meet this younger self and explain the long term damages and effects that artificial sugar causes to your body.

Similarly, you can now also explain the benefits of satiating the sweet tooth cravings with naturally available sugar, and how it benefits your skin, gut and overall mood.

So, let yourself sink deeper and speak to your younger self as if it were your own child.

Longer Pause

And, once you have spoken to the child, we will bring this child with you to the present moment in your life on the count of 3 to 1.

3, 2, and 1…

And now, you are with your younger self in this present moment of your life, fully aware of the benefits of natural sugars and the disadvantages of having artificial sweetened foods or foods loaded with sugar.

In a moment, you will both become one with each other with no cravings for artificial sugary substances anymore, and instead you will now satiate those sweet tooth cravings only with healthy and nutritious food.

Now, imagine your adult self and your younger self integrating into each other, and let your younger self reside in your heart, and see yourself as one - excited to stick to the weight loss plan and achieve your weight loss goal together.

Longer Pause

You are now aware that sweet drinks and sweetened foods with sugar are like poison.

And with this awareness, you are able to spot sugary foods easily and stop yourself from eating and drinking them.

You instead think wisely and choose foods with natural sugars to satiate the craving. This will ensure you continue to make healthy choices while satiating your sweet tooth cravings.

Pause

You are now one with your younger self, and you now satiate your sweet tooth cravings by only consuming naturally available sugar in fruits, and you have now also begun to enjoy having fruits and vegetables as part of your daily diet.

You are also now able to picture yourself at your ideal weight. You look and feel fantastic. You cannot remember the last time you felt so confident and attractive.

You have reached your goal by making these subtle changes to your diet, and by adding daily exercise to your routine.

How amazing does it feel to have achieved this goal?

Pause

Low Carbohydrate Diet

Now, I want you to join me on a fun exercise where we will play a little game using your imagination.

Picture a full platter of freshly cut, delicious, and colourful fruits and vegetables.

Pause

As you take a closer look at the platter, you notice how fresh and delicious the fruits look, and as you begin to smell the fragrance of your favourite fruits, you start to salivate.

Pause

You pick up your favourite fruit, and you take a crunchy bite, and you immediately feel the delicious flavours ooze into your mouth, and you can sense your taste buds dancing with joy.

Longer Pause

There was a time when you had overlooked these beautiful fruits and vegetables, but today you realise the importance and goodness of it. And you have now consciously made the decision to switch to a low carb diet which is another wise decision toward a healthier and active lifestyle.

Pause

You are now fully aware of all the health benefits that come with eating nutritious foods. You understand that it not only helps you lose weight but it also significantly helps you stay mentally alert.

Nutritious food helps you get through the day effortlessly.

A nutritious diet consists of lean proteins, fruits and vegetables, and whole grains, and these foods feed your body with minerals and vitamins which are essential for a healthy body and mind.

It is important to maintain a healthy balance of carbohydrates and proteins as they are an excellent source of energy.

Vegetables and fruits are a great source of fiber which keep your stomach full for longer periods of time.

The darker the veggies, the more nutrients they contain.

With this well balanced diet, you will have beautiful, glowing skin, and an attractive body.

You will be completely transformed, and you are looking forward excitedly to living a life full of confidence, with an active slim body, and clear, glowing skin.

And this is all going to be possible only because you have made these great decisions today.

Longer Pause

Today you are taking your first steps into the universe of healthy and nutritious foods, of eating mindfully, and taking time to nurture your mind and body.

This is going to help you feel fitter, lighter and you will be brimming with confidence.

Pause

Now I want you to imagine all this healthy food entering your body, and nurturing your body with all the essential nutrients.

You now know that a low carb diet provides your body with small doses of insulin which gets stored in the body as good fat, and is a great source of energy.

A low carb diet leaves no room for fat backlog, and it in fact helps you lose weight too.
Now, use your imagination and picture the insides of your stomach, and take a close look at how light and healthy your stomach feels. How happy and clean your intestines feel after you have switched to a healthy and nutritious diet.

Pause

You are now very aware of the advantages of switching to a low carb diet.

A few of these benefits include weight loss, reduction in the fat stored in your body, and high levels of energy.

And with this knowledge, you can now tick off the low calorie, non-starchy, and protein-rich diet as a success.

Pause

From this moment on, you will be eating a healthier, nutritious diet in small portions to keep your stomach and yourself happy which will help you steadily move toward your weight loss goal.

Pause

You are now more mindful of your diet because of which you have embraced protein-rich, low-carb foods, and colourful and fresh fruits and vegetables.

You now consciously take smaller portions of food spread across six meals per day, and you drink at least eight glasses of water.

You are focussed about eating right and exercising each and every day as that brings you closer to your larger goal of weight loss.

Pause

Now, I would like you to pay close attention to the suggestions I am about share with you, and repeat it in your mind

I eat healthy foods (4 seconds pauses)

I eat smaller portions (4 seconds pauses)

I exercise regularly (4 seconds pauses)

I am conscious of my eating habits (4 seconds pauses)

I eat mindfully (4 seconds pauses)

I exercise regularly (4 seconds pauses)

Pause

Self-Hypnosis

Now, observe as you begin to feel a soothing sensation take over your entire body, all the way from your toes to the top of your head.

Imagine your body releasing all tension and worries as it gently falls into a deep state of relaxation and peacefulness.

Pause

Visualise this peaceful, relaxing feeling as it gently moves upward from your toes, to your ankles, lower legs, to your hips, lower arms, elbows, your upper arms and shoulder through to your neck, back, face and all the way up to your head.

Allow your entire body to sink deeply into the surface where you are sitting or lying down, and gently visualise yourself slowly walking down toward the ocean.

Imagine yourself walking down through a blissfully green tropical forest with tall green trees all around providing you with the perfect shade from the sun.

And as you keep walking, you can softly hear the sound of the waves crashing, you can faintly smell the ocean, and you can feel a gentle breeze brush against you which gives you a very pleasant feeling.

Pause

You now begin to see the beautiful turquoise waters of the ocean as you slowly come to the end of the walking path and onto the warm sandy shores of the ocean.

You take off your shoes and sink your feet into the soft white sand. The sand is nice and warm and makes you feel calm and relaxed.

Notice how long and far the beach stretches to your left and to your right, and notice the sun shine glistening off the water far into the horizon.

Observe the water slowly swelling up and forming waves as they come crashing against the coastline one after the other in a very systematic, and rhythmic pattern.
Pause

Now imagine yourself slowly walking toward the water, your feet sinking into the soft warm sand, and as you keep walking, you begin to feel the heat of the sun, and you start feeling very hot.

As you get closer to the water, you feel the ocean mist gently kiss your skin, and as you keep walking, the texture of the sand is now wet and firm.

You feel a wave wash over your feet as it continues to race up the banks, crash and recede back into the sea.

Pause

As you step forward, you feel more and more waves splash against your feet. The coolness of the water gives you a much needed relief from the heat.

The water is clear, clean and pleasant, and you can easily see the surface as you keep walking further into the ocean.

You can continue to walk further if you wish or take a leisurely swim.
You feel a real sense of joy as you spend more time floating in the water, and you begin to feel deeply relaxed.

You feel extremely calm and refreshed.

Now you gently get back on your feet and start walking back out of the water.

And as you gently stroll along the beach, you feel a sense of relief. All your stress and worries have all been washed away.

As you continue to walk back, you notice a comfortable lounge chair and towel waiting for you.

You lay down the towel on the chair, and gently lie down enjoying the sun, the breeze and the waves.

You lay there and enjoy the stillness for a few more moments.

Now, whenever you're ready gently bring your focus back from this visual vacation.

You begin to slowly bring your focus back to your body, noticing the sensation at the sole of your feet, and you feel the weight of your body against the bed.

You feel completely recharged and rejuvenated, ready to return to your day with a refreshed mind.

Now gently open your eyes, and stretch your arms and legs as you become fully alert of your surroundings.

And remember you can practise this visual relaxation anywhere, at any time of the day. And with each practise you will become more and more skilled at effectively refreshing your mind and body.

Protective Sleep

I would like to take a moment here to talk to you about the difficulties you have been facing of late in trying to get some deep sleep. One of the reasons owing to which this tends to happen is when the subconsious part of your mind assumes the role of a protector. That is to say that while a part of your mind may be trying to get you to sleep peacefully, there is a part that is on high alert, as if on the lookout for any threats or events that may possibly occur at night.

Pause

However, this was not always the case, for in the past you have had someone to keep an eye out for you as you slept peacefully through the night. Be it your parents who may have checked in on you to ensure you slept well and were secure, or a partner who slept beside you, or even a pet guarding you or to alert you should the need arise.

Pause

And of late, for one reason or another, somewhere deep in your mind you feel as if the protection you had in the past is no longer there, so you must watch out for yourself on your own. And for this reason the unconscious part of your mind feels the need to avoid sleeping in order to keep you secure.

Let me take a moment here to assure you that there is no longer any need for the unconscious part of your mind to assume such responsibility and stay on high alert through the night. I say this because there is someone else who assumes the responsibility of keeping you safe and guarding you through the night as you sleep -- watching over you, and that is your guide to protect you. It could be an angel or the one you truly believe will protect and watch over you.

Pause

Your guide is someone who has immense love for you. This guide could even be one of those people who were dear to you, who protected you through the night in the past, but may have since passed on. Though they may not be here with you physically, they are watching over you and ensuring you stay safe at all times, especially during the night.

Pause

And though you may, by now have a fair idea of who this might be, it isn't important, because what matters is that there is someone guarding and protecting you at all times, and this someone loves you very, very much. You may not see them, you may not even feel their physical presence at all -- but they are always there, like a warm, cosy cocoon of safety that resides within your heart as you sleep.

I will now be helping you understand and be able to feel the presence of your guide

as they watch over you and protect you.

Start by relaxing your body slowly and steadily, all the way starting from your toes and ankles. Follow the rhythm of your breath -- breathing in relaxation and breathing out any muscle tension you may feel throughout your body. Let this relaxation move up from your ankles, filling up your shins and calves, as it slowly makes its way to settle into your thighs making you feel twice as relaxed and at ease before moving further up and relaxing your waist and lower back. Feel this heavy relaxation settling into your stomach and back, making its way into your chest and shoulders, all the way through your arms and into your fingertips. Breathe in more relaxation and let go of any muscle tension in your neck, jaw, cheeks, and forehead, all the way to the top of your head. that's right, your entire body is full to the brim with this heavy and peaceful relaxation.

Pause

And now that every part of your body is deeply relaxed, visualise yourself standing at the very top of a grand, beautiful staircase that leads you to a place very special to you, making you feel calmer, more relaxed, and sleepier. As you take a good look at this staircase, you notice how safe and relaxing it feels.

You notice the number of steps on this staircase and you can even notice how relaxing it is to know that it leads to a place that is so special to you.

Pause

Slowly begin descending these stairs, counting yourself down with each step. With each step you take, you find a heavy relaxation sinking into you, making you feel calm and safe. The further down you go, the more relaxed you become. Slowly and steadily everything around you begins to feel a little distant and vague, as if everything was slowly fading away with each step taking you deeper and deeper into relaxation. By the time you reach the very bottom of this staircase, you are so deeply relaxed that the world around you would have gradually faded away, leaving you in your special place to relax. This special place could be a pristine sandy beach or a beautiful garden, maybe you find yourself sitting and enjoying the sunset. Whatever and wherever it may be, allow your mind to simply drift away and wander in this special place.

Pause

As your mind continues to wander, you begin to drift with it, into a calming and relaxing feeling. You feel comfortable, as if wrapped in a warm blanket. Drifting further and further, deeper and deeper, feeling more and more relaxed.

By now you are so deeply and heavily relaxed that any thoughts or ideas or images cropping up in your mind barely make it into your conscious awareness, they just float away, leaving you more and more relaxed.

Pause

Maybe at this point you are so relaxed that even my voice seems to have become softer as if coming from quite far away. And in a few short moments, you will find yourself drifting into a short peaceful sleep. And while you may sleep for a short while, you will be able to return to this relaxing hypnotic rest when I speak your name. The moment you hear my voice calling out your name, you will return to this peaceful hypnotic rest, but for now you are slowly drifting into a very calming and tranquil sleep.

As you continue to enjoy this peaceful sleep, you will dream about all the memories that make you feel warm and cosy, almost childlike, filling up your heart with so much love, more than it can carry, so the love fills up your entire body, every nook and corner, making you feel twice as deeply relaxed and brimming with joy.

As this feeling continues to grow within you, you find yourself faced with the realization that you are not alone in feeling all this love and joy and warmth. That out there in a parallel plane of life, there is someone who shares this feeling with you, who loves you just as deeply as you love them. And you soon realise that they are watching over you in a very special way, making you feel so safe and deeply relaxed that you find yourself drifting further and further, deeper and deeper into a state where sleep comes to you with so much ease.

Pause

Soak it all in. Take a few moments here to take in all the love, joy, and tranquility that this moment and this realization brings with itself. Enjoy every bit of this feeling.

That's right.

Pause

And now, from this very moment, you are capable of naturally and easily drifting into a peaceful and relaxing deep sleep whenever you so desire. You are able to find yourself settling into a relaxing hypnotic rest whenever you feel you are ready to sleep. And from there you will drift into your special place, just like right now, and in that special place you will find yourself feeling every bit of the love and protection from your guide. And as your guide will protect you through the night, you will find yourself drifting into deep sleep with ease.

Pause

You are capable of sleeping for as long as you desire, and should you awaken in the middle of the night, you will easily and naturally return to deep sleep by simply tapping into this relaxing state of hypnotic rest.

Relaxing Sleep

Every time you want to fall asleep, you can simply begin by relaxing your physical body in the same way as you have done today. Begin by closing your eyes, taking a deep breath and then scanning and relaxing each part of your body from your toes all the way up to the top of your head.

Pause

You will feel a heavy sense of relaxation sinking into you as you scan your toes and ankles, your shins and calves, going up to your knees and thighs, gently relaxing your hips, your waist, and your lower back as you scan your way up to your stomach and your back, moving to your chest, relaxing your heart, feeling the relaxation building up in your arms and fingers, and as you scan your neck, jaw, eyes, forehead and head you feel absolutely relaxed inside-out.

Pause

Once this heavy sense of relaxation has settled into every part of you, you can picture yourself standing at the very top of a majestic staircase. This staircase leads you to a place that is very special to you. A place where you feel completely safe, at ease, and very very sleepy.

Begin to count yourself down as you begin descending this staircase slowly and steadily. The further down you go, the more relaxed and sleepy you feel. And as you descend through this majestic staircase you will begin to feel the world around you fading away the more relaxed you feel, and this makes you even sleepier. At the bottom of the staircase you find yourself in a very special and safe place -- it could be a garden, a beach, a meadow, or even the mountains, where you can sit or lie down comfortably as you watch the sunset. So let your mind drift and let it take you to this special place. Let go. As you begin to let yourself go, you find yourself surrounded by a warm cosy mist.

Pause

And just like this mist, let yourself drift to where your mind takes you. There is no need to think, just sit back and observe from a distance. Notice the sights and images that crop up through your subconscious mind as they gently float and drift along with you. Softly and slowly, drifting and floating, floating and drifting, slowly and slowly.

As your mind continues to float slowly along with this comfortable and warm mist, you feel deeply relaxed and safe. You feel joy filling you up from within as you continue moving along and drifting with the mist, freely floating. You feel more and more deeply relaxed, sleepier and sleepier than ever before.

Pause

A few moments from now, you will find yourself gently settling into a short sleep. And for now, continue to picture and enjoy this cosy mist settling into this special place around you. Little by little the entire landscape begins to fill up with this mist, so soft and comfortable. The mist starts to become thicker and thicker, making you feel more and more comfortable and deeply relaxed. The thicker the mist becomes, the more at ease and sleepier you become.

Pause

So, let this mist grow thicker and wrap your special place with lots of warmth and comfort. The more you do so, the more you notice how various thoughts, images, feelings, and memories begin to drift in and out of your awareness. You are so deeply relaxed and sleepy that they pass you by without entering your awareness as you continue to focus on the sound of my voice. The more you pay attention to the sound of my voice, the dimmer these thoughts and memories become. They seem to fade away every now and then and you become more and more relaxed.

Pause

You are now completely wrapped up in this warm, cosy, and soft mist that makes you feel so comfortable and relaxed in every nook and corner of your body. All of the thoughts, feelings, and memories have faded so much they almost seem vague. Even my voice by now seems to have become more distant as if it were fading away too, leaving you more and more relaxed and at ease.

Any thoughts that do make their way into your awareness seem to fade away quickly, leaving you more relaxed. And with each passing moment, it begins to get more and more misty, all the thoughts and feelings and ideas fade in and out of your awareness, becoming more and more vague with each passing moment, as the mist continues to thicken, my voice becomes fainter as if coming from further and further away.

Pause

It may seem like my voice is becoming more and more distant, fainter and fainter with each passing moment as you continue to drift further and further. Floating away in the mist feeling more and more relaxed, comfortable, and sleepier. You find yourself drifting further down within yourself, becoming sleepier and deeply relaxed, down into a naturally sound sleep.

Pause

You will only sleep for a short while, and then soon after you will be able to hear my voice calling your name. When you do notice my voice calling your name, you will find yourself slowly coming out of this short sleep and returning to a peaceful state of hypnotic rest.

Pause

You are now drifting deeper and deeper. Everything around you is becoming more and more vague as you drift away into a comfortable sleep.

Pause

Great, from now on you are able to gently float into a restful sleep whenever you desire to do so. You will be able to drift into a peaceful hypnotic rest as you get ready to go to sleep, following which you will find yourself in your special place, being surrounded with a warm and cosy mist, with all your thoughts and feelings fading away slowly as you fall asleep. You can sleep for as long as you desire and wake up easily, feeling refreshed.

Be Healthy

When you are trying to achieve your ideal weight goal, you are not only looking at eating the right food, but you also looking at including at least 30 minutes of exercise into your daily routine.

And as you begin to enjoy this process, it becomes easier for you to achieve your goal.

Staying focussed and motivated about achieving your weight loss goal is very essential in achieving the end result.

Pause

Now picture yourself in the future where you are confident, attractive and healthy, and when you look at your future self, you will feel proud of all the efforts you took to make this possible.

Your focus and motivation to eat right, exercise regularly, and staying positive during the difficult periods has helped you achieve your goal.

And you realise how you continued to grow in confidence with every step you took toward a healthier and happier lifestyle.

Now, think of all the benefits that come with weight loss, and notice how you feel, and note what kind of activities you are looking forward to.

Longer Pause

And as you make a mental note of all the activities you would enjoy, I want you to listen to my words carefully, and repeat it to yourself in your mind.

I am slimmer (10 seconds pause)

I am releasing extra weight (10 seconds pause)

I am confident (10 seconds pause)

I love myself (10 seconds pause)

I am fit (10 seconds pause)

I am excited to lose weight (10 seconds pause)

I am motivated to lose weight (10 seconds pause)

I exercise regularly (10 seconds pause)

I eat well and in smaller portions (10 seconds pause)

Be More Active

Continue to keep a gentle focus on your breath, and let yourself breathe naturally as you drift deeper and deeper into a relaxed state of mind.

And pay close attention to every word I say while keeping an open mind because each and every word is intended with a greater purpose to help you achieve your larger goal.

You are a loveable individual, and from this moment on, you will be confident, and you will be in complete control of your thoughts and actions.

You will be mindful of your eating habits, and you will consciously choose healthier and nutritious food options.

Longer Pause

You will immediately recognize your emotional triggers such as when you are bored or feeling down, and you will be mindful to navigate these challenges in a relaxed and confident manner.

You will engage yourself in physical activities such as walking, running and exercising daily.

You will spend time connecting with your friends, family and loved ones.

You will use constructive methods to unwind or divert your attention by watching light hearted content when you need a laugh, or you will spend time reading a book.

Pause

You will take control of what you eat, and you will reach the ideal goal weight by choosing healthy and nutritious foods.

You will also spend 30 to 40 minutes exercising every day, and this is going to help you lose weight and reach your goal faster.

Pause

You can split your exercise routine into two parts. You could do 15 minutes in the morning, and 30 minutes later in the day or vice versa.

With each passing day, you will slowly feel physically and mentally more upbeat which will give you the energy and motivation to exercise more.

You will look and feel confident, toned, attractive and happy.

And as you progress, you will continue to constantly lose weight and tone up in a healthy manner.

Maintenance Insomnia Relaxation

When we go to sleep at night, we do not really follow a process of falling asleep -- we just do., because we just know how to. Sleep is natural and simple, and a good night's sleep is capable of making us feel refreshed, energized, and rejuvenated and ready to start our day and get things done as we go about our daily living.

However, for some people, this simple and natural course of sleep may get interrupted as they may awaken due to unwelcome and unwanted thoughts cluttering their mind, making it difficult for them to rest and fall asleep or stay asleep. The longer these thoughts linger, the harder it becomes for them to fall asleep.

Pause

The Law of Reversed Effect in Hypnosis, or as we often call it Coue's Law, suggests a reason for this, and that reason being, the more we try to remember or the more we try to do something, the more difficult it becomes for us to remember or do it. So, the more one tries to escape the intrusive thoughts and fall asleep, the more difficult it becomes to do so.

Pause

You may have noticed it too. Perhaps while trying to remember someone's name or even a word to describe something -- no matter how much you try you just can't seem to remember what it was until much later when you are not actively trying to remember it, and it suddenly dawns on you almost out of nowhere!

Pause

The solution? To stop trying and let go. The only way to beat the Law of Reversed Effect is to stop fighting it. This is exactly how we are going to win against the problem you have been experiencing lately -- of awakening in the middle of your sleep, and then trying and trying very hard to go back to sleep.

The solution to this problem, as mentioned before, is to simply stop trying and to stop putting in any effort to fall back asleep. The moment you let go, you will fall asleep just like that. As if it was always that easy and natural.

Pause

Whenever you find yourself awakening in the middle of your sleep, you will simply put away the thought of sleeping from your mind. You can instead think about anything and everything else -- planning for the next day, the things you need to get done, prioritising and deciding what could be done first and what could be done last, or maybe even solving a riddle someone asked you a while ago, or rehearse some activity you were planning to do. You can think of just about anything. You may even get up from your bed and do something else -- perhaps a task you had long been putting off for later. But the one thing you absolutely cannot do is to think of falling asleep.

And soon when the next day arrives, you will wake up to find yourself having slept and slept well. That sleep came so easily and naturally to you, without any effort. You will find yourself surprised at how easy it was, one moment you were planning your activities for the next day, and the next moment you wake up fully relaxed and energised to begin your day after a restful sleep full of sweet dreams that gently lulled you back to sleep.

Pause

From this moment on, the most efficient tool you have is that of letting go. Let go of the perry or the need to fall back asleep any time you find yourself awake at odd hours. Simply use that time to plan and rehearse and reflect on the things that are on priority and need to be done. Complete a few chores if you have to -- anything but trying to go back to sleep. And you will find yourself drifting into a state of relaxing deep sleep without you even noticing it. And when you wake up refreshed the next day, you won't even be able to pinpoint when or how you went back to sleep, but you did, and now you are well rested and free from the worries that no longer hold importance in your life.

Pause

You are now able to remind yourself to remember that you must forget about trying to or even thinking about sleep, for it is something very natural and easy and simple, and it will come to you naturally and easily. Eventually, you will find yourself so adept at remembering to forget about sleep that you will most naturally begin sleeping peacefully every single night without awakening in between even once, only waking up at the regular time the next day feeling fresh and full of motivation to get things done and have a great day -- all because now you are in the habit of getting a good night's sleep every night.

Pause

You can so easily now remember to forget to remember to sleep, and when you forget to remember to go back to sleep, you will find yourself resting through the night in a good night's sleep every time and only awakening the next morning at the scheduled time to get started with your day. Just remember this and you will be fine.

Inner Strength and Power

If you continue listening to every word I say with utmost concentration and enthusiasm, you go into an even intense, deeper, and relaxed state of mind and body. Your imagination is carrying you to a lovely green meadow in your mind, a meadow full of fresh green plants, trees, and hills. The beautiful green meadow is surrounded by lots of flowers in different colors like blue, yellow, red, white, and the ones that are your favorite. Imagine yourself walking through the meadow in a fresh and pure atmosphere.

Longer Pause

You are now looking up at the sky and you see a stretch of the bluish bright skyline with a hint of rays from the sun. It is a beautiful, warm day with a slight breeze that is making you feel like you are in a movie. As you keep moving ahead, appreciating nature's charm, you see a path that leads to a grand beach. You continue walking towards the beach feeling calm and blessed.

Longer Pause

Once you reach the beach you take off your shoes and feel the warm, fine-grained, white sand on the skin of your body. As you start wandering on the sand for few minutes, you find a very relaxing lounge with a bonfire. You get excited and sit by the fire. You take a glance around and you notice there is only you as far as your eyes can see. Gradually you feel a wave of tenderness and realize that even you are sitting beside a bonfire you have a very heavy coat on your body.

You realize that even though you have had it for a while now you have noticed it just now. You reach through the pocket of your coat and you find a small piece of paper in there. The paper has a name written on it of someone that you are not very fond of and someone who stresses you out most of the time. The reason for the stress caused by the person is very clearly mentioned on the paper. You look carefully at everything that the paper reads (get an ideomotor response). After having a glance thoroughly, you crumble the paper and throw it into the fire. You watch the paper slowly turning into ashes, you see the black smoke rise up and disappear in the air.

This is making you happy. You search your pocket one more time and once again you find a piece of paper in it. The paper has a name on it of someone you know and someone who stresses you out most of the time. The paper also points the reasons why this person is the reason for your stress.

Look carefully at everything that it mentions. After reading it you crumble the paper and throw it into the fire. You watch the paper burning and the smoke from it disappearing in the air.

Longer Pause

This makes you happy but a little annoyed as well this time. Once again you decide to dig into your pocket and this time as well you find one. You wonder what is going on. When you pull your hand out from the pocket, you bring a handful of little chits with more names written on it of all the people and circumstances that have troubled, outraged, or have hurt you at some or other point in life. You get angry and throw all the papers in the fire and as each paper turns into ashes, it makes you lighter and happier. You lift your left index paper when all the papers have been turned to ashes.

You feel light as if you're whole body has been released from agony. You feel free as a bird. You then decide to throw your coat into the bonfire as well. You want to experience freedom and don't want any kind of heaviness weighing you down in any way. You close your eyes, take a deep breath in and out and feel calm.

Pause

You now begin to hear a vague sound, something like a waterfall that is far away. You start walking towards the sound, the sound gets clearer when you move towards it, and you then find that it is certainly a grand waterfall with a huge pond of fresh blue water, nothing like you have seen before.

The sound of the water from the fall makes you happy and homely. The place where you can connect yourself with no guilt and opinion, a place that gives you inner strength and peace. Here, if you wish to swim into the water and have pleasure, then you just have to live up to your index finger. Now, you can fearlessly move forward and dive in (give them a few minutes)

Just stand under the fall and try to grab all the natural wonders that surround you. As the fresh, clean and cold water touches your body and flows from above your body to your toes, you feel it is cleansing and taking you away from the insecurities, doubts, and fears contained inside you, especially about your weight.

Pause

You let the water carry away all the negativity that is stored inside you and that goes everywhere you go- from your body far away with the water, let everything go. (Get an ideomotor response when this feels complete to them)

The strength inside your mind and body is rising and glowing. Space that was filled with negativity and bad thoughts is now replaced by happy thoughts and positive energy. You are in love with yourself all over again, you bond much stronger with your inner self this time. Let this feeling sink in and thank the waterfall for providing everything you need to stay happy, calm, and joyful.

(Have them stay with the image as long as you feel it's appropriate, repeating some of these positive words)

It's now the time to remember and thank all the amazing places that you strolled in your mind. Thank the beach, the waterfall, the beautiful meadow for teaching you new things and for bringing positivity and hope in your life.

Suggestions

"Now's the time to make some important conclusions that will adversely affect you."

(Pause)

"With more energy and good vibes, your body is becoming tougher and healthier than it used to be before" (or however they want their body to look and feel)

"You feel great and your body looks perfect"

"Now you only want a healthy diet, you hate sitting idle and you love exercising daily"

"You are gaining more and more confidence each passing day"

"You are happy with everything in all aspects of your existence. You might not realize this at the minute but its completely fine, the more you try, the more suggestions will come your way and will transform you into an amazing way"

Connect with Your Special Place

This is a meditation that is making you feel good about yourself, is going to calm and relax your body and mind, and is going to help you imagine a special place for yourself. This is a place where you are going to feel special and at peace. Therefore, now allow yourself to go into this special place.

It is going to be either indoors or outdoors and is a very special and secure place. I would love you to continue imagining this amazing place. You must become aware of how it feels to be there...

Sense the smell captures the beauty and notices everything that you see.

Longer Pause

Now find a place where you comfortably sit. As you sit, try to feel the place beneath you. Now I am wondering if you could make this place even better and charming. You will feel empowered even just by spending time over there.

Longer Pause

When you sit in your special place you will find yourself at your ideal goal weight.

Longer Pause

Have a strong belief in yourself

You are a very confident woman and you believe in yourself, you are aware of your capabilities, and trust your choices. You have certain qualities that are appreciated by all. Try and recall them as I take a few minutes off.

Longer Pause of 20 seconds

People appreciate you for who you are as a human being and like you for the qualities that you possess.

Now I wonder if you remember your top 5 best qualities. They could either be simple, usual, or unusual, it depends. Just get the knowledge of these.

Longer Pause

What are some of the other reasons that make people like you or drawn to you?

Longer Pause

You are a strong independent woman and a very confident person. As you recall these superb traits that you possess, you feel more confident, strong, and superior.

Confidence in your abilities

You know that you are capable of achieving anything and everything that you put your mind to or get on the path of achieving it.

You are well aware that you can finish any task perfectly and on time with the right execution. And I even wonder if you have a goal that you want to achieve in your mind.

Pause

As soon as you think about the goal that you have in your mind, I would love you to imagine wondering about it and thinking about how to achieve it. You have done a lot, shed off your blood and tears to achieve this goal, now you only have to take the right actions so that it could be achieved with precision and with perfection.

When you recall your preparation it will automatically boost your confidence because you have worked hard and are well prepared for it. And according to the record, if a person prepares well and in advance, is worthy enough to execute it in an even better way and finish it with perfection. Be it any goal, doesn't matter.

The goal could either be eating healthy or exercising regularly. You even know that if you prepare yourself mentally, you can achieve the goal easily and with perfection. You just have to prepare for it with dedication. For example, if the goal is going for jogging or hitting workout sessions, you can go for it by putting on an alarm, keeping your socks and shoes out, and keeping your sportswear out.

As you prepare you to feel confident enough that you are going to achieve this goal. And as you are out to achieve the goal, you will accomplish it. This will boost your confidence to another level and make you into a truly confident woman.

Pause

And from now onwards, you are this super confident, strong-headed, and focused woman. Every time you prepare for achieving something, you are confident enough that you will perform with great dedication and will be at your best.

Longer Pause

You trust and respect yourself which is of utmost importance, people respect you. And as you are thinking about this I wonder if you can press your index finger against your thumb and say the word- confidence with confidence. And if you will notice that if you press them hard against each other your confidence doubles and if you press it harder it triples up.

Pause

This means that anytime you need to feel confident enough in a certain situation or boost it harder, you simply have to press your index finger against your thumb and you will be filled with immense positivity, confidence, and enthusiasm to tackle any situation better.

This makes you confident enough to achieve your goals, confident enough to talk to people around you with assertiveness. With this, you set boundaries that are easy for you, and this, in turn, raises your self-esteem and self-confidence.

Affirmations

1. You enjoy eating raw, fresh fruits and vegetables every single day and savor their flavors. (Pause for 10 seconds)
2. You are motivated to hit the gym and workout regularly(same as above)
3. Your positivity is increasing with your growth and you are becoming more positive as you progress. (same as above)
4. You are now more focused on your daily actions and daily goals(same as above)
5. You can visualize yourself at your ideal weight and all the outcomes and benefit that come with that(same as above)
6. You stay attentive and focused on this weight loss journey that you are going on(same as above)
7. You love the aroma and the taste of this raw healthy food (same as above)
8. You enjoy the taste, flavors, and colors of fresh vegetables and fruits. (same as above)
9. You have started including lean protein and dairy products like skimmed milk in your diet. (same as above)
10. You have even started to enjoy the taste of salads(same as above)
11. You are becoming thinner and thinner day by day(same as above)
12. Your waist is getting smaller, slimmer, and in shape(same as above)
13. You are getting leaner and stronger with each passing because of the hard work that you put in(same as above)
14. You are gaining muscles and shedding off the extra mass that you hate on your body(same as above)
15. You feel strong and confident every single day and this motivates you to do better than ever(same as above)
16. By trusting your body and mind it is getting easier and easier for you to trust yourself. (same as before)
17. Your health is getting better and is improving every day. (same as above)
18. You now can make smaller changes for the highest good. (same as above)
19. You have become more confident, patient and have started to believe in yourself a lot more(same as above)
20. You trust yourself that you are on the right journey, the journey that will take you towards your goal(same as above)
21. You easily let go of the past mistakes that you committed(same as above)
22. You are against emotional eating and you can easily say no to it. (same as before)
23. Weight loss is becoming easier and better for you day by day(same as before)
24. You feel positive, energetic, and enthusiastic after waking up(same as before)
25. Your future is in your hands and you are solely responsible for it(same as before)
26. You have gained more belief in your strengths and capabilities(same as before)
27. You are capable of losing the extra mass off your body(same as above)
28. You love yourself more than before and you take care of your mind and body with the most dedication. (same as before)
29. You are contained with love and brimming with self-care (same as above)
30. You intake foods that are healthy and rich in nutrients(same as above)
31. Your confidence is boosting every day(same as above)
32. You are brimming with confidence(same as above)

33. You trust and believe yourself(same as above)
34. Your self-love and care is increasing every day(same as above)
35. You are now more focused on this journey of weight loss(same as above)
36. You are getting fitter and in shape(same as above)
37. The right choices that you make are sailing you through this journey of weight loss(7 seconds pause)
38. Everyone around you is supporting and applauding you for your sheer dedication and hard work(7 seconds pause)
39. You constantly imagine yourself at your ideal weight, the goal weight that you have in your mind(7 seconds pause)
40. You are mindful of eating healthy and fresh(7 seconds pause)
41. You easily deny the offer of unhealthy food(7 seconds pause)
42. Your body is in sync with your mind and together these two is doing wonders(7 seconds pause)
43. You eat only when you are physically starving(7 seconds pause)
44. You are excited that you will achieve your goal weight and even more excited about how you will maintain it. (7 seconds pause)
45. You are permanently and easily losing weight(7 seconds pause)
46. You are in love with your body and enjoy yourself in this journey that will help you earn your desired body through the hard work that you put in(7 seconds pause)
47. You are shedding off extra mass(7 seconds pause)
48. You are satisfying your appetite by taking the right food in the right proportion(7 seconds pause)
49. You work out daily (7 seconds pause)
50. You are well aware of your eating schedule(7 seconds pause)
51. You like to watch content on weight loss and healthy food every day, it motivates you to do better and better(7 seconds pause)
52. You are excited to work on your mind and body consistently and with dedication(7 seconds pause)
53. Your body and its every cell is getting healed(7 seconds pause)
54. Every day you offer gratitude and wake up with the feeling of gratefulness(7 seconds pause)
55. You trust the cycle of life and even more trust yourself(7 seconds pause)
56. You are well aware of the capabilities of your body and mind(7 seconds pause)
57. Your love for yourself is unconditional and pure(7 seconds pause)
58. You are gracious and compassionate towards yourself(7 seconds pause)
59. You eat healthily and enjoy every mouthful(7 seconds pause)
60. You chew every bite many times and enjoy the flavors (7 seconds pause)
61. You are capable of doing wonders(7 seconds pause)
62. You deserve all the love and care that life has to offer(7 seconds pause)
63. You work out regularly and take care of your health(7 seconds pause)
64. You are filled with confidence and courage(7 seconds pause)
65. You forgive yourself for all the past mistakes(7 seconds pause)
66. You like to stay in the present and are more mindful(7 seconds pause)
67. You know when and how to say no to emotional eating(7 seconds pause)
68. You are conscious about what and how you eat(7 seconds pause)
69. You have daily goals of exercises and eating right in proportion(7 seconds pause)
70. You stuff yourself only when you are actually hungry(7 seconds pause)
71. You enjoy this journey of weight loss(7 seconds pause)
72. You enjoy each day of this journey(7 seconds pause)

73. The result starts to appear soon in front of you(7 seconds pause)
74. Every day you are becoming more confident and courageous(7 seconds pause)
75. You are getting fitter and more desirable with every passing day(7 seconds pause)
76. You are enjoying your life even better by eating healthy and in the right amount(7 seconds pause)
77. You love your body with all your heart(7 seconds pause)
78. You eat healthy food which is rich in nutrients and is of great value(7 seconds pause)
79. You eat fruits and vegetables in different colors (7 seconds pause)
80. You can easily identify the difference between mental and physical hunger(7 seconds pause)
81. You make the right choices about your diet(7 seconds pause)
82. You enjoy each day(7 seconds pause)
83. You are motivated enough to achieve your target(7 seconds pause)
84. You work out daily at least for 30 minutes(7 seconds pause)
85. You get amazed by the progress you see in the mirror(7 seconds pause)
86. You often listen to the saved recordings(7 seconds pause)
87. You have high self-confidence(7 seconds pause)
88. You are worthy(7 seconds pause)
89. You are desirable(7 seconds pause)
90. You are fitter than ever(7 seconds pause)
91. Most often you are in good mood(7 seconds pause)
92. You are happy and full of positivity(7 seconds pause)
93. You allow positive energy to surround you every day(7 seconds pause)
94. You choose to look at the glass half or full daily(7 seconds pause)
95. You are thankful for everything(7 seconds pause)
96. As soon as you get on the bed you fall asleep(7 seconds pause)
97. As soon as you press your index finger against your thumb you feel calm and relaxed(7 seconds pause)
98. You are becoming leaner and fitter(7 seconds pause)
99. You look beautiful and happy(7 seconds pause)
100. You take care of your body beautifully(7 seconds pause)
101. You take immense care of your body (7 seconds pause)
102. You appreciate eating raw fresh fruits every day and love to savor their flavors (Pause for another 10 seconds)
103. You want to exercise every day. (same as above)
104. You are giving positive rays as you progressing. (same as above)
105. You are now more focused on your goals and daily actions(same as above)
106. You can now easily visualize yourself at the weight you always desired, the weight which comes with a lot of benefits(same as above)
107. Stay focused on this journey of fat loss(same as above)
108. You are now enjoying the taste of raw healthy meals(same as above)
109. You are enjoying the taste of fresh fruits and vegetables(same as above)
110. You are now including lean protein and skimmed milk in your diet(same as above)
111. You are enjoying the flavors of salad(same as above)
112. You are becoming leaner and leaner day by day. (same as above)
113. Your waist is becoming slimmer with each passing day. (same as above)
114. You are getting tougher and stronger every day. (same as above)
115. You are losing weight and gaining power(same as above)
116. You feel healthier than before(same as above)

117. By trusting your body you are now able to trust yourself easily(same as above)
118. Your health is upgrading every single day(same as above)
119. You now can bring in small changes for the highest goods. (same as above)
120. You have become patient and you tend to believe more in yourself(same as above)
121. You believe that you are on the right path(same as above)
122. Now you can easily let go of the past(same as above)
123. You are against emotional easting(same as above)
124. Weight loss has become easier for you(same as above)
125. You feel new energy after waking up(same as above)
126. You are the creator of your future(same as above)
127. You are gaining confidence in your fortes and capabilities(same as above)
128. You have the power of becoming an ideal person(same as above(
129. You are in love with yourself even more than before and this is making you take care of your mind and body(same as before)
130. You are blossoming with love and care(same as before)
131. You consume high food rich in nutrients(same as before)
132. Your confidence is on another level these days(same as before)
133. You are confident and believe in yourself(same as above)
134. You trust your worth(same as above)
135. Your self-love and care is accelerating(same as above)
136. You are more focusing on your goal, the goal to reach your ideal weight(same as above)
137. You are getting slimmer and leaner(7 seconds pause)
138. Your ability to make the right decisions is helping you to move further in this game of weight loss (7 seconds pause)
139. Every soul surrounding you is applauding you(7 seconds pause)
140. You constantly imagine yourself being at your goal(7 seconds pause)
141. You are mindful of eating raw and fresh(7 seconds pause)
142. Now you easily deny unhealthy eating habits(7 seconds pause)
143. Your body is syncing with your mind(7 seconds pause)
144. You eat only when you are hungry(7 seconds pause)
145. You are excited by the fact that you will achieve your ideal weight(7 seconds pause)
146. You are getting rid of the fat permanently(7 seconds pause)
147. You love this journey of moving towards your ideal weight, the journey which is leading you to achieve your desired body(7 seconds pause)
148. You are getting rid of the masses (7 seconds pause)
149. You are eating the right amount of food in the right proportion that is required for losing weight(7 seconds pause)
150. You exercise every day(7 seconds pause)
151. You are mindful of your eating patterns(7 seconds pause)
152. You gain knowledge about weight loss and healthy food every day (7 seconds pause)
153. You are enthusiastic about working towards the goal that you have(7 seconds pause)
154. Your cells are getting powered and are healing(7 seconds pause)
155. Every day you wake up for a new start, a new journey(7 seconds pause)
156. You believe this process and have confidence in yourself(7 seconds pause)
157. You trust the journey(7 seconds pause)
158. You are confident enough(7 seconds pause)
159. You are generous towards yourself(7 seconds pause)

160. You enjoy your food and eat mindfully(7 seconds pause)
161. You chew slowly and enjoy the taste(7 seconds pause)
162. You are strong enough(7 seconds pause)
163. You deserve every bit of the love and care that you get(7 seconds pause)
164. You shed off sweat every day and take care of your body(7 seconds pause)
165. You are determined and full of courage(7 seconds pause)
166. You forgive for all the mistakes that you did unintentionally(7 seconds pause)
167. You like to stay mindful in the present(7 seconds pause)
168. You know how to ignore the feeling of emotional eating(7 seconds pause)
169. You are conscious of your eating schedule(7 seconds pause)
170. You have a daily goal of workout and eating healthy(7 seconds pause)
171. You stuff yourself only when you are starving(7 seconds pause)
172. You are enjoying this beautiful journey of walking on the path of being fit(7 seconds pause)
173. You enjoy each day of this journey(7 seconds pause)
174. You see the outcome soon(7 seconds pause)
175. You become more and more confident with each passing day(7 seconds pause)
176. You are getting fitter and slimmer(7 seconds pause)
177. You enjoy eating healthy(7 seconds pause)
178. You enjoy being in your body(7 seconds pause)
179. You consume food rich in nutrients(7 seconds pause)
180. You eat fruits and vegetables in different colors (7 seconds pause)
181. You can identify the difference between mental and physical hunger(7 seconds pause)
182. You choose food wisely(7 seconds pause)
183. You enjoy life to the fullest(7 seconds pause)
184. You are determined to achieve your goal weight(7 seconds pause)
185. You work out every day for half an hour(7 seconds pause)
186. The process encourages you when you notice it in the mirror(7 seconds pause)
187. You listen to the recordings most often and that helps you keep moving in this journey(7 seconds pause)
188. You have high self-confidence (7 seconds pause)
189. You are full of worth(7 seconds pause)
190. You are beautiful and amazing the way you are(7 seconds pause)
191. You are fitter than ever(7 seconds pause)
192. You are in good mood and give positive vibes always(7 seconds pause)
193. You are positive and joyful(7 seconds pause)
194. You like positive energy surrounding you(7 seconds pause)
195. You look at the glass half-full day-to-day(7 seconds pause)
196. You are thankful for this life and all the amazing things that you have(7 seconds pause)
197. Just by three breaths, you fall asleep as soon as you lie down o the bed(7 seconds pause(
198. When you press the index finger by the thumb you feel comfortable and calm(7 seconds pause)
199. You are becoming leaner and stronger(7 seconds pause)
200. You look amazingly beautiful(7 seconds pause)
201. You amazingly look after your body (7 seconds pause)
202. With every passing day you become fitter and healthier (7 seconds pause)
203. You love living every day (7 seconds pause)
204. You look forward to living a healthy lifestyle (7 seconds pause)
205. You are consciously eating (7 seconds pause)

91

206. You are mindful of your eating (7 seconds pause)
207. You love yourself unconditionally (7 seconds pause)
208. You are ready to transform yourself (7 seconds pause)
209. You achieve your daily goals (7 seconds pause)
210. You are mindful of your eating habits (7 seconds pause)
211. You sleep well (7 seconds pause)
212. You sleep on time and wake up fresh and happy (7 seconds pause)
213. Your days are brighter and happier (7 seconds pause)
214. You look healthy (7 seconds pause)
215. You enjoy healthy food (7 seconds pause)
216. You look happy (7 seconds pause)
217. You get compliments from friends and family (7 seconds pause)
218. You appreciate your efforts and your healthy body (7 seconds pause)
219. You eat healthy food (7 seconds pause)
220. You enjoy healthy eating (7 seconds pause)
221. You enjoy the sight and taste of green vegetables (7 seconds pause)
222. You love being healthy (7 seconds pause)
223. You are healthy (7 seconds pause)
224. Each organ is brimming with health and vitality (7 seconds pause)
225. You are attractive in every way (7 seconds pause)
226. You are smart and good enough (7 seconds pause)
227. You enjoy healthy foods (7 seconds pause)
228. Life is good (7 seconds pause) (7 seconds pause)
229. You enjoy your workouts (7 seconds pause)
230. You move your body more. (7 seconds pause)
231. Your body is getting sculpted with every passing day. (7 seconds pause)
232. Your body is more toned (7 seconds pause)
233. People appreciate your efforts (7 seconds pause)
234. You are inspiring (7 seconds pause)
235. You have inspired many already (7 seconds pause)
236. You enjoy living each day (7 seconds pause)
237. You are active (7 seconds pause)
238. You are fit (7 seconds pause)
239. You are positive (7 seconds pause)
240. You are happy (7 seconds pause)
241. You eat smaller portios of healthy food (7 seconds pause)
242. You have fast metabolism (7 seconds pause)
243. You enjoy the taste of fresh fruits and vegetables (7 seconds pause)
244. You drink atleast 8 to 10 glasses of water daily
245. You have a flat stomach
246. You fall asleep easily as soon as you get to the bed for the purpose of sleeping
247. You burn fat while sleeping
248. You are lovable
249. You are getting even more attractive
250. You forgive yourself for all the past mistakes
251. You also forgive others
252. You have high self esteem

253. You are confident
254. You are losing weight with every passing day
255. You are focused on your weight loss journey
256. You pay more attention to the journey than the ideal goal weight (7 seconds pause)
257. You are good enough (7 seconds pause)
258. You have high confidence (7 seconds pause)
259. You are an achiever (7 seconds pause)
260. You take pride in your achievements (7 seconds pause)
261. You eat only when you are physically hungry (7 seconds pause)
262. You do not eat when you are emotionally hungry(7 seconds pause)
263. You believe in yourself (7 seconds pause)
264. Your body is coming in shape (7 seconds pause)
265. You trust your body (7 seconds pause)
266. You trust yourself (7 seconds pause)
267. You trust the process of life (7 seconds pause)
268. You entire body is accepting the new weight loss regimen (7 seconds pause)
269. You are improving in every way , every day (7 seconds pause)
270. You are mindful of what you eat (7 seconds pause)
271. You enjoy your weight loss journey
272. You are the creator of your future. (7 seconds pause)
273. You are in a better space when it comes to food. (7 seconds pause)
274. The choices and decisions you make for yourself are for your higher good. (7 seconds pause)
275. You are no longer holding on to any regrets or guilt about your past food choices. (7 seconds pause)
276. You have accepted your body's shape and you feel blessed for what you have. (7 seconds pause)
277. You have moved away from toxic relationships (7 seconds pause)
278. You accept and acknowledge your strengths (7 seconds pause)
279. You allow yourself to feel good about being you. (7 seconds pause)
280. You have an acceptance for yourself. (7 seconds pause)
281. You are hopeful. (7 seconds pause)
282. You see your future filled with certainly and hope (7 seconds pause)
283. You think of your tropical island every time you decide to sleep 7 seconds pause)
284. Falling asleep is easier than you thought 7 seconds pause)
285. You enjoy your sleep time (7 seconds pause)
286. Your mind knows the importance of sleeping on time 7 seconds pause)
287. You maintain sleep hygiene (7 seconds pause)
288. You do not have caffeine post 5 pm (7 seconds pause)
289. You look forward to sleeping on time every night (7 seconds pause)
290. You are getting mentally stronger with every passing day (7 seconds pause)
291. Life is good with good healthy food and exercising habits 7 seconds pause)
292.
293. You enjoy your workouts 7 seconds pause)
294. You drink plenty of water 7 seconds pause)

Extreme & Rapid Weight Loss Hypnosis: Self-Hypnotic Gastric Band, Guided Meditations & Positive Affirmations for Food Addiction, Confidence, Mindfulness & Healthy Eating Habits

© Copyright 2021 - All rights reserved.

The content contained within this book may not be reproduced, duplicated or transmitted without direct written permission from the author or the publisher. Under no circumstances will any blame or legal responsibility be held against the publisher, or author, for any damages, reparation, or monetary loss due to the information contained within this book; either directly or indirectly.

Legal Notice:
This book is copyright protected. This book is only for personal use. You cannot amend, distribute, sell, use, quote or paraphrase any part, or the content within this book, without the consent of the author or publisher.

Disclaimer Notice:
Please note the information contained within this document is for educational and entertainment purposes only. All effort has been executed to present accurate, up to date, and reliable, complete information. No warranties of any kind are declared or implied. Readers acknowledge that the author is not engaging in the rendering of legal, financial, medical or professional advice.

This book contains 12 guided meditations. The total running time for all the scripts combined will be around 5 hours. Proper instructions have been included for the narrator regarding when to pause and resume the narration. Apart from the twelve meditation scripts, the book has two additional chapters. The first chapter offers some techniques for the readers that they can inculcate in their daily life for rapid weight loss. The second chapter is a guided practice about how to eat mindfully and consciously to help the readers maximise their experience of eating without putting on the extra weight.

The scripts are in the following order:

1. **Effective Weight Loss Techniques** 97
2. **Conscious Eating Practice** 100
  1. Healthy Eating Hypnosis – 10 minutes 104
  2. Getting into your perfect body – 10 minutes 109
  3. Control Craving – 15 minutes 116
  4. A slimmer, fitter you – 15 minutes 120
  5. Health and Wellbeing – 20 minutes 127
  6. Diet Control Meditation – 20 minutes 134
  7. Weight loss meditation – 20 minutes 140
  8. Health and Positivity – 30 minutes 145
  9. Affirmations for good health – 30 minutes 155
  10. Ideal Weight hypnosis – 30 minutes 167
  11. Taming Addictions – 40 minutes 175
  12. Journey to your ideal weight – 60 minutes 183

1. Effective Weight Loss Techniques

We struggle to reach our ideal weight and maintain it. We ask for advices from our fitter and slimmer friends but fail to cope up. And in our seemingly never-ending struggle to lose weight, we wonder if we will ever be able to achieve that perfect body.

What we don't realize is that weight loss is more about mind than about the physical body. When the mind is in control, the body falls in line. To lose weight, you need to manage what you eat, when you eat, how much you eat, and how you eat your food. And all these decisions take place in the mind. You have to program your mind to change how you think about food and choose your food. This book, when thoroughly practiced, will transform your relationship with food forever – obviously, for the better. So, try out all the different techniques and methods at your disposal and stick to the ones you feel are working for you. Again, the weight loss journey is more about the mind than the physical body.

Here are some powerful and effective techniques that you can inculcate in your life to lose weight, reach your ideal size and maintain that ideal size and weight.

1. Do not starve yourself

Many people resort to starving in the name of dieting. That's absolutely wrong. It will have serious implications not only for your physical health but also your mental health. When you are hungry, go and eat. If you starve yourself, your body thinks there is a food shortage and it will begin to store fat. If you starve yourself, you will soon be binge eating. What you must understand is that real physical hunger is completely different from emotional hunger. Physical hunger is natural and gradual. Emotional hunger, on the other hand is subtle. When you feel lonely or upset or maybe when you feel bored, you try to change your feelings with food. You try to improve your mood or maybe just pass the time by eating more food. That's what leads to weight gain. So, eat when you are genuinely hungry. And by being genuinely hungry I mean physically hungry and not emotionally hungry.

2. Don't label food as Forbidden or God-sent

We have this tendency to segregate foods into good and bad. When on diet, we want to eat only the ones we feel will help us get slimmer while ostracizing the items we think will make us fatter. One thing about naturally thin people is that they eat chocolates, cheese, anything that is fried and oily, and all the forbidden food. But they don't eat in excess. So, taste everything but don't indulge in excess. Many people these days go on diet and they forcefully eat food that they don't like and then they feel like they are missing out on life's pleasures. Because as soon you decide this food is exactly you should not eat, it becomes all you could think about. So, the lesson is that don't label certain food items as forbidden and others as god-sent. Being slim and fit is more about your eating habits than about the food.

3. Eat Mindfully

Whenever you eat anything, eat it with full awareness. Some people have the tendency of thinking about food all day long, except when they are actually eating it. They eat the food as fast they can. Research study has shown when we eat slowly and mindfully, we eat less. So in future when you eat, be mindful throughout the act of eating. Cut the food, put it into your mouth and put the knife and fork down and chew the food very slowly, about fifteen to twenty, and savour it. Feel the flavours, the texture, the taste. And be mindful and conscious when you are eating. Do not be in any hurry to finish your meal. Just be mindful, and eat slowly. And when you eat, just eat. Do not do any other activity while you are having your food because if you watch TV, or listen to a radio or you are online using social media, you will end up eating more. So, when you are eating, focus on the food and nothing else. Enjoy your meals and savour them to the fullest.

4. Stop eating when your stomach signals that it's full

When you think you are satiated, stop eating. If you keep eating your food really fast, you ignore the signal that your stomach gives to your mind that it is full. So, you keep eating and eating and eating and end up feeling bloated after the meal. And then you will feel the guilt of indulging too much. We add extra fat because we eat more than our body needs. And it's not the fault of our body our mind that fails to listen to the alarm signal of the stomach because you were eating too fast. But when you eat slowly and mindfully, you will listen to the signal of being satiated and you will stop. And if you feel hungry later, and by hungry I mean physically hungry and not emotionally hungry, you can eat again – slowly and mindfully.

5. Balance is the key

Don't go to the extremes. Plan a sustainable diet and exercise routine. You are working hard so that you not just reach your ideal weight but also keep it. Extreme methods may give results initially but that won't last for long. Having a balanced approached, just like other things in life, is essential in losing weight and maintaining your ideal shape. Fasting one day one overeating the next day not only negates the benefits of eating less but also upsets the digestive system. Similarly exercising to the extremes for a week and avoiding gym for the rest of the month won't do any good to your physique. Begin with a simple and practical diet and exercise routine and then gradually increase the intensity. The key is to be regular with your routine and for that you need to have a balanced approach all throughout.

2. Conscious Eating Practice

Welcome to this mindfulness practice to improve your experience of eating. Before we begin, I must tell you that this is not a regular meditation where you sit still in a meditative posture with closed eyes. Today, we will meditate will eyes open. Meditation has no specific definition. So, the act of being present in the moment is also a form of meditation. And doing each activity consciously and with full awareness is akin to meditating.

Before we start, I want you to keep near you an apple or any other fruit in a ready to eat condition. You can peel off the skin of the apple and cut it into smaller pieces if you want to. If you want to have any other fruit, that's fine. If you don't have any fruit in your home right now that's also completely fine. You can pick any eatable for this practice. It can be salad, sandwich or a chocolate. Don't bother about the nutrition content of the food. This meditation is about how to eat mindfully rather than a lecture on what to eat. So, when you are ready and have food near you, I want you to relax your body with three deep breaths. Breathing in through the nose and out through the mouth. Breathing as deep as you can be aware of your breaths. Follow the breath.

Focus and breathe in. Hold. And Release.

Breathe in. Hold. And Release.

Breathe in. Hold. And Release.

Very good. Now breathe at your normal pace. Maintain a focus on the movement of your breath. Stay fully aware of the present moment.

[10 seconds]

Connect with the physical sensations in your body. Can you feel the sensations of hunger? How hungry are you? We often fail to acknowledge hunger as a signal for the body to recharge itself. We rather associate hunger with emotions, with pleasures, or even with time. We simply don't eat when we are hungry because we don't feel the feeling of hunger.

So, now I want you to feel that feeling of hunger and then answer. How hungry are you right now? On a scale of zero to ten, with zero being not hungry at all and ten being starving for food.

[5 seconds]

Can you get a sense of how hungry you are? And keep in mind hunger is not all about food. You might be hungry for something entirely different than food. Listen to the language of the body.

[5 seconds]

And then assessing your food as if it is the first time you are seeing it. It will be the first time you will eat something. So, bring that sense of freshness in your thought. Set aside all notions and tastes. Look at the fruit or whatever your food is as if you are seeing is for the first time and will be consuming any type of food for the first time.

[5 seconds]

So, what does your food look like? Does it look appealing? What colour is it? Notice the shades of colours intermingling with one another. Now pick up the food and hold it in your hands. How does it feel? Notice the weight of the object. Is it heavy or light? Does it feel cool, warm, smooth or rough? Can you feel the texture? Raising the object up to the ear noticing any sounds generated by the object. Perhaps squishing or tapping the object. Opening up to sounds or lack of sounds you hear. If you notice the mind wandering away or if your analytical mind is saying that all this is appearing weird, that's okay. It's the natural tendency of the mind to over think. Just come back to the present moment. Come back into the physical senses as you explore this object.

[5 seconds]

Now bring the object towards the nostrils, noticing any sense of smell. How does your food smell?

[5 seconds]

Then as you are ready, slowly taking your first conscious bite. Tasting, savouring, chewing slowly and investigating the experience of eating. Letting your intention be on the taste and the changing textures and the sounds of eating. You might even close your eyes to really tune in. You are aware of chewing, swallowing and then pausing between each bite even putting your utensil down and taking your mindful breath. And be sure to eat each bite thoroughly. Taking the time to taste the food. May be even the taste satisfaction, knowing that no two bites are exactly the same. How much flavour is there? It might be different that what your mind is telling you.

[5 seconds]

You may also notice swallowing the object tracking it all the way down the throat, and into the belly.

[20 seconds]

And from time to time pause to investigate your hunger and your fullness. You might discover that you are tired of eating the food you have chosen, or you might discover that you are no longer hungry even though there is still food on the plate. Give yourself the permission to stop or continue based on what you discover.

Maintain a moment to moment awareness of your direct experience. Savouring your food means taking time to choose food that you really like, to choose food that honour your taste buds and your body.

[10 seconds]

Savouring and becoming fully present for the experience of eating and the pleasure it can bring. Whenever you have notice that your mind has wandered on to the future or the past bring it back to the experience of eating, tasting, savouring. Taking time with your meal, pausing between bites. Being interested and curious about changing sensations and textures and tastes. Pausing to assess taste satisfaction. How satisfying is this bite? You might notice physical changes in yourself.

[10 seconds]

Now that you have a choice to how much to eat and when to stop eating.

[10 seconds]

Continue with this mindful meal breathing, eating, savouring, pausing and checking in. And this is not a one-time activity. Make this conscious eating a habit. No matter wherever you are and whatever you eat, eat consciously.

Thank you! Have a nice day!

1. Healthy Eating Hypnosis – 10 minutes

Get comfortable in a nice sitting position. Take a moment to settle into the body.

[5 seconds]

Bringing some softening to the shoulders. Make sure the crown of the head is lifted. Sensing into the body as a whole. Feel more and more relaxed. Feel the energy here that is holding you. Inhale slowly and then slow steady exhale through the mouth.

[5 seconds]

If the nasal passages are open allow the mouth to gently close. Feel more and more relaxed. And sense the flow of the air in the nostrils. Noticing the temperature, perhaps any coolness or warmth.

[5 seconds]

Inhale deeply allow for slow comfortable exhale. Feel more and more relaxed. Perhaps bringing the slight extension to the exhale without forcing.

[5 seconds]

Intuitively know of the count if that is helpful to link in the exhale. Even out any edges of the breath, exhale slow and comfortable, smooth. Allowing the breath to be in its rhythmically natural flow. Feel more and more relaxed.

[5 seconds]

Keep the breath calm, steady and sustainable. Consider what needs to be brought in and brought forth, steady the mind and shift the attention to the body.

[5 seconds]

Allow the breath to travel to the base of the body. Feel the stability. Feel the support. And now feel the breath supporting the support. Your breath is such a wonderful tool. Use your breath as your anchor. Feel your breath spreading throughout your body and relaxing you. Be aware of the movement of the breath.

[5 seconds]

Feel the rise and fall of the chest.

[5 seconds]

Inhale, sense the lift and expand the chin. Exhale the softening. Relaxing your shoulders. Releasing any strain or tightening in jaw.

[5 seconds]

Listen to the beating of your heart. Feel any vibrations or tingling in the hands.

[5 seconds]

Now feel the whole body breathing.

[30 seconds]

Now that you are completely relaxed, we are going to work on your subconscious mind. So take three deep breaths. In through the nose and out through the mouth.

[10 seconds]

Relax and breathe at your normal, rhythmic pace.

[5 seconds]

We are now going to tap into your power of creative visualisation. I want you to go back down your memory lane and think about a time when you were feeling really bored. Think about a time or situation when you were doing something that made you feel extremely bored or even disgusted. Take your time and recreate that feeling of boredom as strongly as you can in your mind.

[5 seconds]

Now, I want you to feel that feeling of boredom and hold on to that feeling for a while.

[5 seconds]

Now replace that feeling of boredom with the act of eating. Go on. You will notice that your subconscious mind is getting into action and replacing feelings of disgust and boredom with the act of eating. The activity that originally bored you is being replaced with the act of eating. Let that feeling and connection sink deep within you. The more you think about it and connect it, the more deeply will it ingrain in your subconscious mind. And that is very important. Because once the message is received by your subconscious mind, half the work is done. Then your subconscious mind will make sure you make the right decisions and take corrective measures to achieve your goals. So feel that connection. Once again, replace the feelings of disgust and boredom with the act of eating and let that connection sink in deep.

[5 seconds]

Now, picture yourself sitting at a dining table. You can see at the table piles of food. Food that are full of fat and oil and are very unhealthy but seem delicious. In normal conditions it would be very difficult to resist eating such food. So you begin to eat. You take the first few bites and you find the food tasty. But soon, your interest in the food fades away very quickly. You take a few more bites and you begin to feel tired.

[5 seconds]

Your subconscious mind is making your body realise that overeating is not good for you. You enjoyed the first few bites. Your subconscious mind knows that eating this much is fine. And after those first few enjoyable bites, you begin to feel disinterested in the food. You don't feel like eating more. You feel tired.

[5 seconds]

Now, even the thought of eating more than required by your body makes you feel disgusted. But at a deeper level, you know that this change is positive for your health and wellbeing. You have always wanted it this way. Enjoying the first few bites of a food and then stop eating it. But you always used to over eat and that resulted in weight gain. You gained weight because you never knew when to stop. But now you stop at the right time for you to get slimmer and fitter. Now, you feel so good. Just a few bites and you already feel satiated. You don't want to eat more. Just the thought of eating more than a few bites makes you feel tired.

[5 seconds]

From this day onward, you will only as much food as is required for your body as a fuel. Just after you have eaten that small quantity that is enough for you, you will feel the urge to stop eating and leave the table.

You will focus far less on the activity of eating as it will appear very boring to you. You will from now on focus more on more positive activities that feel so much interesting to you. These activities like exercising, running, cycling, swimming, or playing outdoor sports are very fruitful for your health. The more you exercise or do any other physical activity that keeps you fit and healthy, the more you enjoy doing that exercise. All the fitness related things now excite you. You feel yourself spending more time taking care of your body. You arrange your life in such a way that you spend substantial time in physical and health restoring acivities.

[5 seconds]

From this day onward, you will be eating food that is good for you, food that is healthy and nutritious. You will indulge in activities that will help you lose weight and get into proper and ideal shape and size. You will be far less interested in the act of eating and so much more interested in activities like exercising, swimming, jogging, and doing physical activities that keep you fit. You indulge more in meditation and yoga that help you stay calm and focused. You will everything that will take you closer to your goal of achieving and maintaining your ideal weight and size.

[5 seconds]

The positive feeling that you have right now, I want you to visualise this positivity in your heart chakra, located in the centre of your chest. Feel your heart chakra in bright pink colour. Know that all the positive changes are already within you. All you have to do is tap into your heart chakra to access these positive thoughts and ideas. Stay with this healing positive light for a while.

[30 seconds]

Now I am going to count the numbers form 1 up to 5. With each number that I count you feel yourself becoming more and more alert. You will also feel yourself becoming more and more positive and in control. At the count of 5 you will then open your eyes feeling completely refreshed and alert.

1

2

3

4

And 5.

Gently open your eyes. Feel refreshed, feel positive, feel focused. Namaste!

2. Getting into your perfect body – 10 minutes

Start by sitting in a comfortable position. Make sure your back is straight. Relax your shoulders.

[5 seconds]

Take a moment to settle into this space. Allow your eyes to gently close. Allow the hands to rest comfortably.

[5 seconds]

Consciously release tension from neck, relax the shoulders moving them down away from the ears.

[5 seconds]

Now, bring a gentle awareness to your breath – the inflow and the outflow.

[5 seconds]

The inflow and the outflow.

[5 seconds]

Try to notice the quality of your breath. Is it shallow or deep? Is it rough or smooth.

[5 seconds]

Observing, just observing the breath without any attempt to change it in any way.

[5 seconds]

Now allow your attention to drop into your body. Feel your body. Feel the space around your body.

[5 seconds]

Feel the outline of your body.

[5 seconds]

Now feel your physical body.

[5 seconds]

Feel the weight of your pelvis, hips, on the chair or the mat or the sofa or bed.

Bring your awareness to your belly. And feel the movement with each inhale and exhale. Feel the rise and fall of the belly.

[5 seconds]

Take a couple of deeper and fuller breaths now. Inhale and feel the lift of your belly, as it expands away from the spine. And as you exhale notice the belly release.

[5 seconds]

Continue to take ling and deep breaths.

[5 seconds]

Inhale and feel the sides of the ribs expand. Exhale sense the ribs move in towards the mid line.

[5 seconds]

One more deep and long breath. Inhale and the belly rises. Exhale gently and it falls back.

[5 seconds]

One more deep and long breath. Inhale and the belly rises. Exhale gently and it falls back.

[5 seconds]

One more deep and long breath. Inhale and the belly rises. Exhale gently and it falls back.

[5 seconds]

Allowing your shoulders to relax, jaw released. Resting here with your breathing. Couple of more inhale and exhale. Inhale and exhale. When you are ready allowing your breath to settle in and come more naturally. Encouraging stillness in your body.

[5 seconds]

Breathe at your natural pace. Maintain a gentle awareness of the movement of your breath – the inflow and the outflow.

[30 seconds]

If your mind wanders, gently bring it back to your breathing.

[30 seconds]

Now, once again bring a gentle awareness to your breathing. Follow the breath as it journeys in and out of your body.

[10 seconds]

Notice your chest as it rises and falls with every breath you take.

[5 seconds]

Notice the air moving in and out from your nostrils as you gently breathe.

[5 seconds]

Look into your heart and imagine that a bright pink light is radiating from your heart. It's all the love that you feel in your heart for the people in your life and for the goodness in your life.

[5 seconds]

Now visual this pink light expanding and getting bigger and bigger and it covers your entire torso and your back. And now it expands and covers your shoulders and hips and arms and legs and your face and hands and feet.

[5 seconds]

And as it expands and spreads to your different body parts, it activates the power of loving kindness and gratitude and compassion that you deeply associate with. This light is so pure, so powerful. It is the light of love, the light of healing. It is the light of empathy and compassion and all things positive. You feel the light and all the goodness in all your cells and organs and your entire body.

And you realize the healing potential of this powerful healing light. Today, it will heal all that you want to heal. And you request the healing light to work on your health and fitness. You request it to heal you and make you slimmer and fitter.

And you see the light travel to your digestive system and filling it with its pure, healing light. From now on, you will digest your food properly and absorb all the nutrients and nourishment without accumulating the unwanted fat.

[5 seconds]

And you feel so grateful. Your digestive system is a miracle, it has an intelligence of its own. From now on, it will work to make you slimmer and fitter. It will absorb all the goodness from what you consume. And you say to your digestive system that you will from now on consume only those food items that are healthy. You will drink more and more water so that your digestive can work efficiently and digest your food properly.

[5 seconds]

From now on, you will give your digestive system better food, healthier food, and more nutritious food. You will eat food mindfully and you will chew every bite at least twenty times. You will show gratitude for your food and for your digestive system.

[5 seconds]

Now this bright pink light of healing travels to your internal organs to remove all the layers of fat source around your mid section.

[5 seconds]

Visualize the light targeting and removing specific areas of fat in and around your belly, removing fat from your waist and from your entire abdomen region.

[5 seconds]

Anywhere in and around your midsection, you can send this healing light to cut, cleanse, and remove the extra layers of fat that have been troubling you. Use your imagination to guide this light.

[20 seconds]

And now visualize sending this light to any fat in and around your hips and thighs and legs. Request the light to help you get rid of this extra unwanted fat. And you see the light doing its magic.

[5 seconds]

And is this light removes the extra layers of fat from your hips and thighs and legs, you can feel a sense of relaxation in these areas.

[5 seconds]

Now you see this light travelling to your shoulders and removing the extra fat.

[5 seconds]

And then to your biceps and removing the extra, unwanted layers of fat from there.

[5 seconds]

And moving down to your forearms. You can see the bright light cleansing all the unwanted fat from all over your arms.

[5 seconds]

And now visualize this light moving on to your neck and removing the unwanted fat. And then moving up and removing the extra fat from your chin.

[5 seconds]

Visualize this bright healing light shaping your jaw muscles and removing the extra fat. And then your cheeks and around the nose.

[5 seconds]

You can visualize this healing light removing the extra layers of fat from your forehead.

[5 seconds]

Now, you can send this healing light to any part of your body that you think is having some extra, unwanted fat. Take your time and cleanse the fat.

[30 seconds]

Now visualize yourself at your ideal physique and your fittest body. You are now rid of all the unwanted fats. Visualize yourself standing in front of a mirror and behold the image of a perfect you. Visualize yourself in your favorite cloths. You look so good. You feel so confident. Feel the confidence that comes with this perfect body. And thank the pink light of healing for working its wonders for you.

[30 seconds]

Now, taking a long, deep breath and come back to your body. Gently moving your fingers and toes. Relaxing your shoulders. And coming back into the room you are in.

[5 seconds]

Rubbing your palms against each other.

[5 seconds]

And bringing your hands to your eyes and gently massaging your closed eyelids.

[5 seconds]

Now join your hands and bring them to your chest with your thumbs touching the heart chakra.

[5 seconds]

Feel grateful for this healing meditation. Namaste!

3. Control Craving – 15 minutes

Welcome to this meditation for controlling your craving. We will begin to make you feel comfortable and then move on the visualization part. So, find a comfortable place. Close your eyes or keep them open, softly gazing down and breathe in and out of our nose and two fill our stomachs up with air instead of your chests. This allows us to be even deeper and most common breath.

[5 seconds]

So as we begin place your hands gently over your stomach or your mid-section. As we take a breath together, breathing into your nose, just notice the feeling of filling your stomach up with air, holding it at the top and then slowly letting it go. As we are doing this deep breathing your pace might be different from mine, but just know that's ok. Whatever pace you need to breathe out, is ok right now as long as you are having yourself try to extend it as slowly as you are able to. Together on count of two, to do some breaths. Then try to take some on your own. So breathe in through your nose two, three, four, hold and slowly out 2, 3, 4, 5 and in 2, 3, 4 hold and out, 2, 3, 4, 5. Now you can do even slower now, in 2, 3, 4 hold, out, 2, 3, 4, and 5.

[5 seconds]

Now take some deep breaths on your own. Really noticing and imagine your stomach expanding with air, holding it at the top and then letting it fall gently and relaxed. As you take your next inhale, noticing what the air feels like as it enters your nose. See if you let your exhale; relax all the muscles in your body as the air leaves. End with 2 more guided breaths slowly in 2 ,3,4, hold and out ,2,3,4,5 and in ,2,3,4 hold and out,2,3,4,5.

[5 seconds]

Now we will begin progressive muscle relaxation together. We will be relaxing our bodies starting from our head and scanning all the way down to our feet. Focusing on relaxing every muscle in our inner body to try to send common messages to our brain. As we do this you might notice tension in your body, you might notice tightness, tingling, when you encounter that see if you can just allow yourself , you have that sensation be there. Knowing that it feels okay to that sensation and it's okay to feel the discomfort, allowing it to be there.

[5 seconds]

Begin with the deep breath in through the nose, 2, 3, 4, hold and out, 2, 3, 4, 5. Start by as we scan our body from the top, we will start with the muscle around our eyes, around our eyebrows. As you exhale see if you can allow those muscles to just relax. Feel more and more relaxed.

[5 seconds]

See if you can move down to your jaw, noticing any tension there, and allowing the muscles in jaw to relax. Feel more and more relaxed. As you scan down to your shoulders to your neck, notice any tightness there any places where you are holding, tension or discomfort and as you exhale with your breath, see if you can allow your shoulders to feel heavy and move down towards your back. Feel more and more relaxed.

[5 seconds]

As you scan down your arms, notice that position your arms are in, are you holding your arms tensely. As you breathe out let your arms falls gently and heavily wherever they are resting. Feel more and more relaxed.

[5 seconds]

Now scan down to your hands, noticing all the little muscles in your hands. Let your hand to just gently fall as they are. Noticing heavy relax sensation. Now focus on your chest, your stomach, noticing how they move with your breaths. Noticing any tightness or discomfort you feel there. Allowing it to be there. Knowing it's okay and as you exhale, just allowing that little section of your body to feel heaviness and peace.

[5 seconds]

Now scan down to your hips and thighs. Noticing the strength and ease, areas. Noticing any discomfort or tension as you exhale just allowing the muscles in your legs to release to feel heavy and scanning down to your calves and your ankles, letting them fall heavy and relaxed.

[5 seconds]

Taking a deep breath into your nose and out. Noticing on your feet and noticing any sensation there. There might be tingling in your toes, tightness in your ankles. It's okay to feel these sensations you have. As you take a deep breath in letting your feet relax and exhale, letting them feel heavy. Notice over all sensation in your body. Feeling relaxed, feeling at peace.

[30 seconds]

Now we will work on your cravings. I want you to think about the food which you are out of control around. It may be a chocolate cake or a pizza or anything. Think about the desire you have and rate your desire and scale from one to ten. With number ten being the most and number one being the least. Now think about the food you really think you are really disgusted about. The thought of which makes you go yuck or it is too awful to think about. It might be anything, a broccoli or any food that really disgusts you. So now take a compulsion for the food which you crave. And the repulsion you have, the food that disgust you. Put them together and you will notice that one will cancel out the other. Close your eyes and imagine biting into that food which you really like, the craving food, chew in your mouth as you chew it notice that the food that awfully disgusts you. If it's a chocolate cake, you bit a chocolate may be you taste something which disgusts you. So mix the two tastes together in your mind. The food you feel so tasty that compelled to eat and the food you are awfully disgusted by.

[5 seconds]

Put some hair from barber's shop into the mixture and carry on chewing that food that you really feel really compelled to eat, with the food you feel awfully disgusted by.

[5 seconds]

Make sure that the food you disgusted by is very, very strong. Taste the textures, taste the hairs. Mix them together. Swallow both of them down.

[5 seconds]

Now think about the food you felt compelled to eat and your desire from the scale of 1 to 10, it should be lot lower by now.

So, the next time you have this craving, remember to repeat this exercise.

4. A slimmer, fitter you – 15 minutes

Lie down and relax. Let the arms and legs stretch out. Find a comfortable position. Close your eyes.

[5 seconds]

Take a deep breath in. and let it go.

[5 seconds]

Take a deep breath in and let it go.

[5 seconds]

One more time, Take a deep breath in and let it go.

[5 seconds]

Let your breath return to its natural rhythm.

[5 seconds]

Do a scan through your body to help you bring your focus gently to different parts of yourself and relax a little bit deeper. So you don't have to move anything as far going through just bring your attention to the different parts of yourself. See if there is any tension that you are holding there. I want you to release that tension and let it go.

[5 seconds]

Bring your focus gently to your toes. Noticing each of your toes individually allow yourself to feel each toe. Letting each toe relax.

[5 seconds]

Bring your focus gently to the bottom of your feet. To the tops of your feet.

[5 seconds]

Bring your focus gently to your ankles, to the backs of your calves. Noticing the contact with the surface underneath you and allow yourself to feel supported.

[5 seconds]

Bring your focus gently to your shins. Into your knees, bring your focus gently to the back of your thighs, noticing the contact with the surface underneath you. Bring your focus gently to the fronts of your thighs. Expand your focus to include your entire legs to tips of the toes, all the way up to the body at the hip.

[5 seconds]

Allowing your legs to relax completely. Letting go.

[5 seconds]

Bring your attention to your lower belly and how it moves as you breathe in and breathe out.

[5 seconds]

Bring your focus gently to your waist. Now to your lower back. Bring your focus gently to your upper back. Noticing the contact with the surface underneath you.

[5 seconds]

Bring your focus gently to your lower ribs. Noticing that how they expand when you inhale and then contract as you exhale. Bring your focus gently to your chest, noticing how it moves when you breathe in and breathe out. Bring your attention to your shoulders, allowing your shoulders to relax. Letting go of any tension, any stress they may be holding.

[5 seconds]

Bring your focus gently to your upper arms, and into your elbows. Bring your focus gently to your forearms. And to your wrists.

[5 seconds]

Bring your focus gently to the palms of your hands and now into the backs of your hands. Bring your focus gently to your thumbs, noticing each of your thumbs individually. Notice where they are, are they touching anything or if they are expanded in the air.

[5 seconds]

Bring your focus gently to the other four fingers of the each hand. Noticing each one individually and allowing each finger to relax. Expand your focus gently to include your entire arms. From the tips of your fingers, all the way up to they meet the body to the shoulders. Allowing your arms to relax completely, Letting go.

[5 seconds]

Bring your focus gently to your neck. Into your jaw, letting go of any tension. Bring your focus gently to your back of the head. Noticing the contact with the surface underneath you.

[5 seconds]

Bring your focus gently to the point between your eyebrows if they were to cross your third eye point. Expand your focus gently to include your entire head and then expand it further to include your entire body. And if any part of your body feel requires attention, be free to go back to it now.

[30 seconds]

Now with your eyes closed, I want you to try to focus on your Third-eye located in the middle of your eyebrows.

[5 seconds]

Relax, let go, just breath. You are here today to relax and focus on the healthier version of you. So let's start by taking three deep breaths and imagine you are breathing from the heart space.

The single eye of the heart this is the very powerful manifesting point within the body. So gently inhale and exhale slowly from the heart space. Inhale and exhale.

[5 seconds]

Inhale and let it go. Breathe in and out. Breathing fully in and let the air gently escape out.

[5 seconds]

Now let the breath find its natural rhythm. Feel the breath slowly expanding your abdomen and the chest on the inhale and when you exhale just let the breath go naturally.

[5 seconds]

Remember to breathe from the heart space. Breathe in and out, allow the breath to fill your confidence and the sense of purpose. And gently exhale out that does not serve you.

[5 seconds]

All your anxieties and stress – just let them go with the out breath.

[10 seconds]

Now imagine, you are looking at your true authentic healthier slimmer self, who cares deeply about your health, your physical appearance and your true happiness.

[5 seconds]

I want you to bring in to your mind the qualities and the characteristics about yourself that you value and appreciate so much. Take your time. Be as detailed as you can.

[5 seconds]

Now visualize yourself floating into that authentic self. Begin to engage all your senses. Begin to gaze down at your feet, your legs, your torso, and your arms. How do you look? How does it feel to be your true authentic slimmer self? Feel the feeling. Be your true authentic self.

[5 seconds]

You may experience a sense of happiness and joy that you haven't experienced before. Now see yourself walking around. Walk with full confidence. How does it feel being the healthier and more confident you?

[5 seconds]

Notice the details very, very clearly. Be as detailed as possible. Notice everything. Feel the feeling. Get into the minor details. Where are you? What kind of peoples are around you? What are you doing? Focus on every detail. And most of all focus on your feelings. How do you feel?

[10 seconds]

Focusing in on even more details now. What kind of cloths are you wearing? Be very specific. Take your time to think about your cloths. Feel the cloths on your skin. Feel how perfectly they fit onto you. How do you feel? What's your hair like? See yourself now very vividly, moving around with ease and grace and remarkable confidence. Wherever you go, whoever you meet, people all over are impressed by your transformation. They are mesmerized by this confident version of you.

[5 seconds]

Visualize this in as much more detail as it's possible. The more vivid, the more real that you make it, the more effective it will be. How do you feel?

[5 seconds]

So take a few moments to enjoy experience in your authentic fitter, healthier, slimmer true self.

[5 seconds]

Feel and be the person you really are. Before all your leading believes of how you should look and who you be and feel those wonderful positive emotions. Let those feelings ride into your past space. Take a few more moments, enjoy.

[30 seconds]

Breathe in and gently exhale out. The sense of confidence the real you. Remember you create your own reality by simply focusing upon it. Visualizing but most of all feeling it. Take a nice deep breath.

[5 seconds]

Remember that everything starts out with visualization. This is how all creation takes place. Always be grateful to be you. Now feel these words right into your heart space. Experience them willing to be your entire being, compassion, empathy, kindness, light, forgiveness, beauty, happiness, contentment, abundance, authentic you. These are words to remember anytime you are face with down.

[5 seconds]

Deep within you, you know that your true self wants those changes in your life – experience, compassion, kindness, respect and beauty. To make the change happen you have to feel as if it has already happened. The process will be natural and gradual and you will enjoy every step of your journey. So, keep believing. Keep visualizing. And keep achieving.

5. Health and Wellbeing – 20 minutes

.

Lie down in a comfortable position of rest.

[5 seconds]

Loosen up your body. Relax any areas of stress. Feel completely at ease.

[5 seconds]

Now use your senses and become an observer of yourself and your surroundings. Just observe and do not interfere. What do you hear? Just observe and listen. Do not interfere. Do not judge the sound. Do not call it music or noise. Do not label it. Just let it be. Be just an observer.

[5 seconds]

Do you smell anything? Just observe your sense of smell. Do not judge. Do not label the smell.

[5 seconds]

What do you feel on your skin? Do not label the sensation as harsh or soft. Do not judge. Just observe.

[5 seconds]

Gently breathe in a breath of relaxation and release.

[5 seconds]

And again and release.

[5 seconds]

As a quiet observer, consciously observe your left foot. Notice that you can feel the body alive energy in your foot without touching it. Allow your attention to move your energy to upwards, to the calves of your legs. And to your knee, to your hips and buttocks. Feel completely relaxed.

[5 seconds]

Relaxing the stress as you go and gently breathe in up breath of relaxation.

[5 seconds]

Now as quiet observer, consciously guide you inner attention to your right foot.

[5 seconds]

Allow your attention to move the energy to upwards to the calf of your leg and now up to your knee. Feeling the energy to move upward to your hips and buttocks. Relaxing the stress and as you go.

[5 seconds]

Now tighten up and hold the muscles of hips and buttocks, tight now release, release the stress and again tighten and hold and now release.

[5 seconds]

Let all the tension go , release and feel the peaceful relaxation flowing through your body. And gently breathe in up breath of relaxation. And Release.

[5 seconds]

Do it again.

[5 seconds]

Now as quiet observer consciously guide your inner tension to your stomach area, your solar plexuses. Gently breathe in up breath of relaxation. And release and again.

[5 seconds]

You feel so safe. So relaxed. Release any tension you may feel in your stomach area. Guide your attention and energy upward to your heart. Feel the warm sensations, a peaceful relaxation. Feel relaxed. Allow the loving warmth to spread to your shoulders, to your neck, and throat. And gently breathe in a breath of relaxation, And release. And again.

[5 seconds]

Now feel the energy in your left hand. Allow that energy to move up to your left elbow. Coming up into the shoulders, the neck and the throat. And gently breathe in up breath of relaxation and release. And again and release. Feel relaxed.

[5 seconds]

Now feel the energy in your right hand. Feel it move upward to your right elbow, coming up energy flows into the shoulders. The neck and the throat , joining with the rest of the energy. Feeling the relaxation and again gently breathe in up breath of relaxation and release. Again breathe and release.

[5 seconds]

Now allow your attention and energy to flow upwards into your nose, your ears, your eyes, into your forehead and now to the top of your head, into your highest energy center. Your loving and relaxed connection to the world. Consciously experience the stillness of the moment, the quietness of the mind. Feel your body , experience the warm peaceful relaxation.

[5 seconds]

Observe yourself as being loving ,peaceful and relaxed space. A relax space rather than something stressful in it. Observe yourself as the powerful trusting space, the trusting space rather than something anxious in it.

[5 seconds]

No matter what happens observe yourself as to be free this space, to be the space. Rather than that which happens in the space.

[5 seconds]

Now come let us stay in this relaxed, calming and peaceful state and gently breathe in a up breath of relaxation, and release and again.

[5 seconds]

Stay here. Just observe. Do not judge. Do not label. Just observe.

[1 minute]

As you are lying down. Imagine that the support of the floor is rising up to meet to the weight of your body. Now, you feel safe. You can now can relax and let go. You know that you are fully supported.

[5 seconds]

Flow with your mind the rise and fall of your breath and let every exhale be an opportunity to be relaxed a little more.

[5 seconds]

As you take a few more breaths, just imagine that you are lying somewhere. A clearing has been laid out for you. It could be somewhere you have been before or somewhere you would like to go with a sense of being on holiday. Or you could completely make this place up in your mind.

[5 seconds]

And in this clearing there are blankets and cushions and everything you need to be completely comfortable and to relax. You are present in here and now but also on a holiday in the clearing. And the weather is just perfect. Picture yourself at the age you are today in the cloths you are wearing and really visualize yourself in perfect health on your physical level and your spiritual level, and your emotional level. Visualize perfect health on a creative level and on a mental level. Perfect on every level.

[5 seconds]

And as you look at that image of you in an optimum health, turn up the brilliance and the colour of that image and bring that image closer and closer to you.

[5 seconds]

Closer and closer to you and until you merge with that image.

[5 seconds]

You might initially notice some resistance within you to be in that part of that picture of perfect health. So acknowledge that resistance. Be nonresistant to the resistance, being nonjudgmental and totally accepting and acknowledging all the emotions that come up to you, when you practice this idea of merging with perfect health.

Accept this resistance. This is also important. You realize that visualization is different from reality. But your subconscious mind knows that reality is a manifestation of what we visualize. So, it important that you shed that resistance and embrace the image of that perfect version of you. Because this is your reality in making. So, slowly and gently, accept the image.

[5 seconds]

Focus back on that picture and again turn up the brilliance, turn up the colour and bring it so near that you merge with that image comfortably and easily. Relax. Visualize it happening effortlessly.

[5 seconds]

Let the relaxation of being in perfect health in a clearing on a holiday as you let the wave of relaxation move through you like a tide. Moving down through the jaw, through the body releasing and then releasing. Relax. Feel it softening and relaxing the tongue, softening and relaxing the neck, relaxing the chest region, relaxing the heart. Now feel the belly softening and relaxing. The pelvis muscles softening and relaxing away from their bones, down your legs and deeper.

[5 seconds]

As you stay here, stay in this feeling of ultimate rest and relaxation. Feel at present. You may feel that there is even a deeper shift like a tide that has gone down past your feet. And maybe you feel a tide moving up slowly through your body like a beautiful wave of energy which is carrying a blue wave of health all the way through your body. The blue wave of health through the soles of your feet and the ankles.

[5 seconds]

Feel it moving through the bones in you shins and skin of your legs. Reaching up to your knees.

[5 seconds]

Moving this tide of health, this wave of health back to your waist raising and falling with the tide.

[5 seconds]

Moving up into your shoulders, lapping into your neck and your arms receiving the tide , past your head.

[5 seconds]

Allowing this powerful tide to wash over you, gently. Full of this blue wave of optimum health and for healing.

[5 seconds]

Washing over every cell in your body as you lie here enjoy that sensation of the knowledge of perfect optimum health inside you.

Send some gratitude to your body for all the work it does, sometimes it's difficult to send gratitude to areas that you have struggled with. Now see if you can direct that gratitude at deep real gratitude to those parts and acknowledge the work that your body is always doing to help itself.

[5 seconds]

Feel this wave of relaxation and healing all over your body. Feel it recharging and refreshing your entire being. It gives energy to your image of your perfect self. That image of your ideal self, keep that image in your mind whenever you sit to eat. That image is now etched in your subconscious mind. Your subconscious mind know what to eat and how much to eat to make reach that ideal weight and size and maintain it too. So, keep that picture in your mind. Your subconscious mind will nudge you to exercise more often. It will guide you to stay away from unhealthy foods. It will help you overcome cravings and addictions. Your subconscious mind will take care of everything. All you have to do is keep this image of your ideal version in your mind.

6. Diet Control Meditation – 20 minutes

Lie down. Loosen up your body. Get comfortable in your bed. You can use a blanket to make yourself cosy and comfy. Take your time to adjust your body.

[5 seconds]

And be gently aware of your breath.

[5 seconds]

With each breath that you take, perhaps you can feel your body relaxing a little bit more. For this exercise, we are going to concentrate on the individual parts of your body. Learn to choose a part and to tense that part up. Just for few seconds and then what we are going to do is to relax that part entirely. For this exercise, focus all your attention on your right foot. Now inhale and at the same time clench all the muscles in that right foot as hard as possible for 5 seconds, 4, 3, 2, 1 and exhale and release all the tension as you allow all the muscles in the right foot to become loose. Let it relax.

[5 seconds]

Move your awareness to your right lower leg. Focus all of your attention on your right lower leg and inhale and same time clench all the muscles in that right lower leg as hard as possible for 5 seconds, 4, 3, 2, 1. Then exhale and release all the tension.

[10 seconds]

Now all of the muscles become loose and relaxed. Now we are going to proceed up to your entire right leg. Inhaling and tensing for 5 seconds, 4, 3, 2, 1. Exhaling and relaxing your entire right leg.

[10 seconds]

Moving your attention to your left foot. Inhaling and tensing for 5 seconds, 4, 3, 2, 1... Exhale and release any tension.

[5 seconds]

Now to your left lower leg.. Inhale and tense for 5 seconds, 4, 3, 2, 1. Exhale and release any tension.

[5 seconds]

Now your entire left leg. Inhaling and tensing for 5 seconds, 4, 3, 2, 1. And relax. Exhaling and relaxing your entire left leg.

[5 seconds]

Now focus your right hand. Inhale and tense that right hand for 5 seconds, 4, 3, 2, 1 exhale and release any tension in your right hand.

[5 seconds]

Now to your right forearm. Inhale and tense that right forearm for 5 seconds, 4, 3, 2, 1 exhale and release any tension. Now your entire right arm. Inhale and tense that right arm for 5 seconds, 4, 3, 2, 1... exhale and release any tension in that entire right arm.

[5 seconds]

Now it's time for the left hand. Inhale and tense your left hand for 5 seconds, 4, 3, 2, 1... exhale and release that tension in your left hand.

[5 seconds]

Now your left forearm. Inhale and tense that left forearm for 5 seconds, 4, 3, 2, 1... exhale and release any tension.

[5 seconds]

Now your entire left arm. Inhale and tense that left arm for 5 seconds, 4, 3, 2, 1... exhale and release any tension in your left arm.

[5 seconds]

Now to your abdomen. Inhale and tense for 5 seconds, 4, 3, 2, 1... exhale and release any tension in that abdomen.

[5 seconds]

Now to your chest. Inhale and tense that chest for 5 seconds, 4, 3, 2, 1... exhale and release any tension in that chest. As we focus now on your shoulders and neck. Inhale and tense for 5 seconds, 4, 3, 2, 1... exhale and release that tension.

[5 seconds]

And now we move to your face. Inhale and tense muscle in that face for 5 seconds, 4, 3, 2, 1... exhale and release any tension anywhere in that face.

[5 seconds]

Allow all the muscles in your entire body to come loose and relax.

[5 seconds]

Be in the this state of complete relaxation for a while.

[2 minutes]

We have this naturally ability that we always know when we have had enough food. Our stomach give a signal to our brain that it is full. So, we know when we are satiated and content with the food we are eating. It's so natural and happens every time we eat without fail. And the signal comes every single time we eat. The purpose of eating is to absorb the energy to work through the day. But as we move through life, we tend to forget why we are actually eating. So instead of filling our stomach with enough fuel, we eat unmindfully and tend to overeat. We ignore the signal our stomach gives to our mind and continue eating out of sheer habit. And when we ignore the signals, we eat more, expanding our stomachs and gaining weight. And as our weight increases, our self confidence dips. We feel lethargic and develop low self-esteem. We are afraid to go out and socialise. We avoid meeting our old friends. We fear they might notice that we have gained so much weight. So we make excuses. And our self-confidence keeps on dipping lower and lower. But now you have decided to turn things around. Change will come for sure. And for that you are going to change your eating pattern. And that's not very difficult if you consider this.

Have you ever wondered that small babies have so much smaller tummies than us and they eat so less? And as a person grows older, the stomach expands and that only means that they want to eat more. And this results in weight gain. This means that there is a direct connection between the size of the stomach and the quantity of food we consume. So, I want you to now imagine yourself getting younger and younger. Imagine your physical body going back to the age of ten, nine, eight, now five, and perhaps two years. So when you were two years old, your stomach was so small and you ate so much less than you do now.

And as you listen to this audio, your subconscious mind is connecting with the two-year-old you and is becoming one with the feeling of eating less. Your subconscious mind knows it all. It is activating the feeling of having the stomach of the two-year-old you. So, in your current state and physical body, you have a small stomach. That means you want to eat so much less. Your subconscious mind knows this.

I want you to bring this feeling in your body now. This feeling of having a really small stomach in your body. You have a small stomach that feels full and satiated after eating a very small quantity of food. Feel it deep inside you this feeling. You take in a small quantity and you feel full. This will help you lose weight and shed the extra fat on your body.

You feel content and satiated after eating a small meal. You eat only as much as you feel hungry and that is a very small amount since you have the stomach of a small baby. And when you are served more food, you say no to it. You can only take in small quantities of food now. And since you take in so less, you don't put on more weight. You release the extra weight, the extra layers of fat from your body.

[5 seconds]

And you visualise yourself sitting on a dining table. In front of you is a plate full of food. You see the plate and wonder if you could eat this much food since you have such a small appetite now. And you begin to eat – slowly. You take the first bite and chew it properly. And you chew it mindfully, savouring the bite, enjoying the flavours. You chew the bite for about twenty times.

[5 seconds]

And you take another bite and chew it properly for about twenty times. You notice how good the food tastes now. And you don't feel the desire to eat fast. You enjoy every bite, every flavour.

[5 seconds]

After a few bites you feel satiated. You realise that your small tummy has had enough food and is now full. And this happens every time. Now whenever you eat, you get the signal when your stomach is full. And you stop eating. Your subconscious mind has received the message that your stomach is now very, very small. And it can eat only very little quantities of food. And this little food gives you full energy that is required to get you through the day.

So, imagine yourself with a very small tummy, going about your daily routine with full energy and enthusiasm. And when it's time to eat, you consume so less because you have a small tummy. You feel satiated with small quantities and you begin to go about your daily routine with full strength and energy.

[5 seconds]

Your tummy is getting smaller and thinner and fitter. With each passing day, you are becoming fitter, healthier and more active. You can notice your body getting to the desired shape and size. You can feel the transformation. You can feel yourself brimming with confidence and zeal. This is the life you were meant to live. And your subconscious mind knows it. It has taken in from this audio all that it needed to take in. You can now rest. So, enter the states of deep, deep relaxation.

[10 seconds]

I am going to count you down a night of healing, inspiring, and healthy sleep...

Ten

Nine

Eight

Seven

Six

Five

Four

Three

Two

And one.

7. Weight loss meditation – 20 minutes

Sit in a comfortable position. Take three deep breaths.

Breathe in through the nose and out through the mouth.

[5 seconds]

Very good. Again in through the nose and out through the mouth.

[5 seconds]

And one more time; in through the nose and out through the mouth.

[5 seconds]

Relax and breathe at your comfortable pace. Maintain a gentle focus on your rhythmic breath.

[20 seconds]

Now I want you to bring your awareness to your physical body – your entire physical body. And now move your focus to the connection of your body with the surface beneath you. Be aware. Just feel the connection as precisely as you can. And feel the connection of your bottom with the surface beneath you. Again feel that feeling that as precisely as you can. Be aware. Be fully aware. And notice how it's little different on the left side compare to the right side. Now bringing your awareness to the up to your nose, feeling the breath as it enters and exits the nostrils. All the way in and all the way out. Feeling the breath as it travels up and down inside of a nose. Be fully aware of the moment.

[5 seconds]

You might notice a difference in temperature in the air on the in breath and he air on the out breath. Feelings what happens at the end of the out breath is there a pause for a moment. So feeling that the turning at the end of each breath. Be aware. Noticing how it varies from breath to breath. It's okay, that's part of it. Just noticing that and bring your awareness back to your breath again and again.

[5 seconds]

This is the best way to notice the behavior of your mind. Whether it's busy or quiet, agitated or relaxed, concerned with the particular topic and however it is its just fine. Just bring it back again and again.

[5 seconds]

Now following the breath down in the belly, feeling the rise and fall of your belly, with the in breath and the out breath. Be aware. As we follow the breath into the different parts of the body this is the beginning of the organic body scan.

[5 seconds]

Noticing the quality of the breathing in the belly. Whether it's deep or shallow, tensed or relaxed, smooth or jerky, and allowing it to be without trying to fix and change anything. Be aware. Allowing is one of the key elements of mindfulness. Just feeling how the breath is in the belly. Allowing it to be getting it of own way.

[5 seconds]

Noticing the sensations on the skin as you breathe in and out. Noticing any sensations inside the belly. Any tingling, any fullness.

[5 seconds]

And be particularly interested that how the sensations change over time and with the breathing. And as our awareness becomes more subtle, we can notice smaller and smaller changes. As we notice change, we can let go often things to get fix. As we change they change by themselves.

[5 seconds]

Feeling the breath going into the belly. Notice how it goes down towards the bottom without trying to push in. Just feeling how far it goes.

[5 seconds]

Very nice. Now relax and breathe at your normal relaxed pace.

[5 seconds]

And maintain a gentle focus on your breath – the inflow and the outflow.

[30 seconds]

Now, I want you to imagine that in front of you is a version of you who is just a little bit lighter than you are right now, just a few kilograms lighter. When you can see that you close a little bit looser, float into that you, that's a bit lighter. See through the eyes of you, lighter, slightly your thinner self and feel slight lightness, feel inside yourself. Now from this point, imagine yourself a few kilograms lighter even thinner. Take a moment to imagine that you.

[5 seconds]

Look how move, how your cloths are lighter and looser on you. Then float over and into that thinner you. Feel how it feels to be thinner and lighter. How your cloths feels differently. And how you feel about yourself having lost some weight. Then from this place, imagine even thinner and lighter you. Look how you move, look how your posture is, you cloths are even more loosely on you.

[10 seconds]

Then float over and into the thinner you. See through the eyes of your thinner self. Feel how good it feels to lose even more weight. How your cloths fit so loose! How you got even more energy and you feel good about yourself. Feel the feeling. Things are going in the right directions that you have always wanted them to go.

[5 seconds]

Next imagine even thinner you. You have lost even more weight. You really see how the cloths are even loose on you. Then float over and into the thinner you. Feel the feeling. Feel how good it feels to be this light, to have lost even more weight.

[5 seconds]

Now you feel to be in more in control of your life. See through the eyes of your thinner self. Feel the feeling. Feel how good it feels to be in your body, to be even lighter than you were before. Isn't that fantastic? Let that get into your subconscious mind so that your subconscious mind knows that you want to gradually lose weight and keep the weight loss. Your subconscious mind knows exactly what to do. So just relax and keep visualizing and following the instructions.

[5 seconds]

Then from this place, imagine even lighter you. You just lost even more weight. And look that how you stand, how the cloths fit really loosely now. And float over and into that thinner version of you. See through the eyes of your thinner self. Feel the feeling. Feel that how good it feels to lost this much weight. Isn't that fantastic? How good you feel in this right now?

[5 seconds]

Then from this place, visualize an ideal and perfect you. You have the ideal weight, the ideal size, the perfect skin. Everything about you is just perfect. Isn't that fantastic? And now float into that ideal you.

[5 seconds]

See through the eyes of your ideal self. Feel the feeling. Feel that how good it feels to have this perfect body and this ideal weight. Feel the confidence. How good does it feel?

[5 seconds]

This feeling of being at your ideal weight and size, you can stay in this feeling for a while. And the more you stay in this feeling, the more you become the ideal version of you. So, you can stay in this feeling for as long as you want to.

8. Health and Positivity – 30 minutes

This meditation is best practiced in a lying down position just before sleep. So, adjust yourself into a comfortable position. Close your eyes. Let your body relax. Loosen up your joints, loosen up your muscles. Relax your jaw; relax your shoulders; soften your stomach. Let your whole body relax.

[5 seconds]

Be aware of your breath. Breathing in through your nose and breathing out through your mouth. That's all you are going to do right now. Just focus on your breath. Nice deep breath into your nose and breathing out through your mouth. Taking the breath nice and deep as you breathe in, focus on filling the lungs, stomach all the way down to your legs, all the way down to your toes. So the breath is going all the way through your body and then release.

[5 seconds]

Take a nice and deep breath in to your lungs, your stomach, down your legs, all the way down to your toes. Hold it and release.

[5 seconds]

Resume in a normal breath now. You can let go of any thoughts from your day so far. Let the thoughts come and go. You don't need to attach with the thoughts. Don't give the thoughts any energy. Just allow the thoughts to drift away, just like they have been drifting away like a wave in the ocean. As they come in, you acknowledge them and then you let them go out to the tide, let them go out on the wave and release the thought.

[5 seconds]

Do that with any thoughts that come to mind in this meditation. Don't fight them just allow them to be present be aware of them and then release them.

[10 seconds]

Right now we are going to take all of our focus and attention down into your feet. Think about the bones and the muscles in your feet. Just try them mentally acknowledge that sensations that you are feeling in feet, you may find a tingling sensation, you may feel warmth in the feet or the feet may feel cold.

[5 seconds]

Just put all of your focus and attention right there on your feet and tell your feet to relax. As you breathing in your breath in relaxation as you breath out you start to release any tension, any stress, anything in the body that don't need to be, you exhale and let go.

[5 seconds]

Breathe in relaxation and breathe out and release tension.

[5 seconds]

Starting to get really comfortable. Feel your body to become more relaxed.

[5 seconds]

Allow that relaxation feeling that you have in your feet and any kind of tingling sensation, allow that to build, get stronger and slowly move up into your ankle.

[5 seconds]

All the while just breathe and relax.

[5 seconds]

Thinking about the bones and the muscles in your ankles, moving up into your calf muscles and lower legs. Allow the lower legs to just relax. Allow those muscles to just let go and relax. Breathe and allow the body to sink deeper and deeper.

[5 seconds]

Moving up into your knee, and the bones and the muscle sin your knees and see them letting go and relaxing deeper and deeper.

[5 seconds]

Think about your thighs, and the strong muscles in your thighs. And allow those thigh muscles, just like an elastic band to tightly round up. Imagine the thigh muscles being released so they can become softer and longer. Become heavier and heavier, very relaxed.

[5 seconds]

Moving on to your hips and the bones and muscles in your hips.

[5 seconds]

At this point in your relaxation, involve your mind. Take your mind and your body on a very peaceful relaxing journey. Think about relaxing your heart slow your heart down and allow it to relax at a very comfortable pace.

[5 seconds]

Relax your lungs, your intestine all of your organs working perfectly well, everything is happy, everything is healthy. You can be at peace and feel relaxed.

[5 seconds]

Relax your shoulders, your chest, the muscles across your chest. Notice as you breathe in and then release the breath.

[5 seconds]

Relaxing the muscles on the back of your neck and across your shoulders, breathe and let them get warm, let them get softer.

[5 seconds]

Let your whole neck and shoulders relax.

[5 seconds]

Take that relaxation sensation and allow it to slowly flow down to your shoulders, down into your elbows.

[5 seconds]

Trickling slowly down into your wrists.

[5 seconds]

All the way down to the very tips of your fingers. Your arms are now very relaxed.

[5 seconds]

Now focus on your head, your heavy head. You have to carry and hold up all day right now you can just let go, release your head. Allow your head to sink deeper and deeper. And relax.Now you can just enjoy the fact that you can just let go and release and completely relaxed your head. Now you can notice that your whole body is very, very relaxed.

[5 seconds]

Start to get the sensation that you could just float away up into the clouds. Your legs, your arms, your torso, your head everything is so relaxed. You feel completely weightless. Allowing your body to rest. And relax. This is very easy as it takes no effort at all to start to fly slightly higher and higher up so that you are looking down in the grass, looking down on the trees.

[5 seconds]

Rising up so you can to see the children are playing in the park. Allowing yourself to completely let go and keep rising higher and higher.

[5 seconds]

Notice how your body is starting to feel this very strong feeling of complete freedom. Completely open to its surrounding no weight no worries no stress, just you completely relaxed. Floating higher and higher up now so you are floating right there in clouds. And relax.

[5 seconds]

As you lay here in the clouds this is this highest we need to go today. Everything that you need is right here with you in the clouds. Feel the complete peace that you feel throughout your whole body as you float up here in the empty sky. And relax.

[5 seconds]

Just breathe, enjoy and relax. Know that here in this place the mind the body and your spirit are completely aligned. Here you can see the reality of your life and know no matter what is happening in your life currently, it will be always there to be managed and accessed in the morning. Right now here in this moment, all that you should do is let it go. And relax.

[5 seconds]

You still have breath, you still have life, you still have body, and you have your health see that as your abundance see your problems as something that you can fix later. So relax.

Right now you know in your conscious and sub conscious mind that there is nothing that you can do in this moment. Right now all you have to do is relax.

[2 minutes]

You can be to be on a specific diet to feel your best or because of some sickness you have. Or maybe you are trying to lose weight. But on a reason you are eating healthier, it can be hard. And now this meditation is going to help you to help you remember why you are eating healthier and to help you to hold on to that feeling. It can be so hard, especially if you eaten certain foods for your whole life. Even you eat healthier, makes you feel better and you know that your brain can still revert back to what you have eaten for the most of your life.

[5 seconds]

We are going to work on remembering those good feelings you had for eating well and taking care of your body in a way that feels best for you. All those good feelings that you want to have by eating well and taking care of your body.

[5 seconds]

So let's begin by imaging yourself, feeling how you want to feel for eating healthy or imaging yourself at a time where you were eating healthy. So just picture yourself, during that time when you are feeling good. How do you look? Or how did you look? This isn't necessarily about weight. It's more just about feeling good and how feeling good? And how do you think you look when you were feeling your best? And more importantly then how you looked when you felt that you have eaten healthier? How do you feel when you picture yourself this away?

[5 seconds]

I am sure that you look and feel really good in your own eyes. Because how could you not? You are working on taking care of yourself and in a way that is so perfect. And your body needs you to take care of it in this way. And I want you to feel that feeling all over your body and let that feeling just sink in.

[5 seconds]

Now I am going to help you to move that feeling to all throughout your body.

[5 seconds]

We are going to start by imagining this good feeling to appear in a white ball of energy sitting right above the top of your head.

[5 seconds]

Now I want you to imagine an opening, starting right at the top of your head. Now imagine a ball of energy, slowly opening the entering.

[5 seconds]

Now imagine that the ball is spreading out and moving all throughout your body. It's starting to fill that air in your entire face and your jaw.

[5 seconds]

And then the energy is filling down, filling your neck, and slowly moving down, filling your whole chest and then down filling both of your arms.

[5 seconds]

It's moving down filling your whole stomach. And down through your hips. Down both to your legs all the way down to your feet.

[5 seconds]

Now that white pure, good energy is filling your whole body. And it's swirling all around.

[5 seconds]

This is the energy of how it feels when you eat your healthiest.

[5 seconds]

When you take care of yourself in a way that you feel your best. When you continuously listen to your body and make the best few choices for you. Just feel that feeling keep swirling all throughout your body. That good and beautiful feeling. Feel that feeling.

[5 seconds]

And as it swirls throughout your body, you are also pushing out the energy that may be telling you that you can do your best. You are allowed to feel your best.

[5 seconds]

It's also pushing out any energy that might be telling you it is okay to eat things that don't make you feel good. That energy is not helping you to feel your best. So right now all this good energy swirling around and moving that bad energy out and only allowing space for the good feelings you want to feel, from eating healthy and listening to what our body's need from us. There are only good feelings. There are only good feelings.

[5 seconds]

So I want you to feel this feeling for a few moments.

[5 seconds]

Just feel this good energy swirling all over throughout your body and just pay attention to anything comes out of you. It's normal in this time to receive these messages or things may be you shouldn't be eating in order to remain feeling, this good feeling. Feel this good feeling.

[5 seconds]

Or may be messages that are helping you to keep this good feeling. Be aware of this good feeling. So go ahead and just feel this feeling for the next few moments.

[2 minutes]

You are now able to spend time in conscious about what you eat. Not necessarily how much you eat, because remember we all need food to live. Just really be conscious about what you eat.

[5 seconds]

Absorbing what really makes you feel your best and eliminating what doesn't make you feel your best.

[5 seconds]

There are definitely occasions where that happiness is perfect may be you are spending time with people you love. May be you are just taking time for you. Just as long as you recognize that this can be your everyday. Hope your food makes you feel better every day. You will enjoy healthy foods. And those foods you need every day. When you can always come back to the healthy foods because you better not eat something that doesn't make you feel good. From now on, you will enjoy healthy food that will nourish you without adding fat. And you will be repulsed by the unhealthy foods. You will automatically make the right choices for yourself.

[5 seconds]

Now repeat after me, "I consciously eat in a way that makes my body feel good. I consciously eat in a way that makes my body feel good. I consciously eat in a way that makes my body feel good."

"I am at the peak of my health and fitness, and I will maintain that level of health and fitness. I am at the peak of my health and fitness, and I will maintain that level of health and fitness. I am at the peak of my health and fitness, and I will maintain that level of health and fitness."

9. Affirmations for good health – 30 minutes

Sit or lie down in a comfortable position. We will first be relaxing your body to prepare you for this amazing affirmations meditation for good overall health.

[5 seconds]

Let's begin by softening your entire face. Gently roll your shoulders down and away from your ears. Connect with your breath as you begin to follow your inhalations and your exhalations.

[10 seconds]

We are now going to travel through our bodies, relaxing our bodies from head to toe. But start with the first top crown of your head. Feel a sense of relaxation at the top of your head.

[5 seconds]

Relax your forehead, relax your eyebrows. Relax the space between your eyebrows.

[5 seconds]

Relax your thinking mind.

[5 seconds]

Relax your eyes, your cheeks and your nose.

[5 seconds]

Feel the breaths as it travels into your nostrils. And then feel it as it exhales through your nostrils.

[5 seconds]

Relax your mouth, relax your chin, and then separate your jaw ever so slightly, especially if you have the tendency to clinch your jaw.

[5 seconds]

Even allow your tongue to rest. Let it float in between the upper and lower pallets of your mouths.

[5 seconds]

Feel a slight smile coming of the outer corners of your lips as your entire face begins to relax. Take a moment to visualize yourself to beautiful, soft and tension free face.

[5 seconds]

Relax your neck, the front the sides and the back of your neck.

[5 seconds]

Relax your shoulders releasing any wave your sub conscious is carrying. Relax your upper arms, your lower arms, relax your elbows, your writs, your hands, relax your fingers and your finger tips.

[5 seconds]

Take a breath in from the tips of your fingers travelling up to your arms and shoulders and then exhale relax the center of your chest, middle of your spine as well.

[5 seconds]

Inhale fully and deeply into the center of your belly, expanding outwards and then slowly exhale and then relax your belly.

[5 seconds]

Relax all the internal organs of your body, knowing that everything is working more efficiently more than a few moments ago and trusting in this process that we can quite see with our eyes.

[5 seconds]

Relax the middle of your spine. Relax your lower back. Soften and relax your buttocks. Your pelvic region and your hips.

[5 seconds]

Relax both of your legs and just feel the muscles no longer gripping the bone as they do when you walk and move, but letting go and being relaxed.

[5 seconds]

Relax your knees, your shins, and your calf muscles. Now relax your ankles, your feet and each of your toes.

[5 seconds]

Take a breath from the tips of the toes travelling up your entire body touching each and every part with this invigorating energy.

[5 seconds]

As you come up to the crown top of your head, feel the breath turn over and then begin to exhale, cleanse your body of any toxic or negative thoughts any things you have said that you wish you could take back or any that just feels like a baggage to you.

[5 seconds]

Exhale it down the body, sending it to your toes.

[5 seconds]

And now I want you to imagine that you are standing on a shore of a beautiful body of water.

[5 seconds]

Watch the waves that they go out from the shore, take away that you have released. Feeling lighter making room for more fresh and pure air energy to enter your body once again for next breaths.

[5 seconds]

Inhale once again to the tips of your toes all the way up to the very crown of the head, touching all parts of your body with this breath, with this peaceful energy.

[5 seconds]

As the breath turns over at the crown send it with anything you are holding on to, like to let go off. Send it down your body and up through the toes.

[5 seconds]

Once again picture yourself standing at the shore that expensive body of water that each wave carry what you have released out deeper and deeper.

[5 seconds]

Watching that you have released that again to the vastness of the beautiful body of water. Rid yourself of that energy that might have toxic or negative feelings. Feel lighter and freer and more relaxed and at peace now that you have made space for the purest of the fresh breath and energy to enter your body. Relax in this space for a while before we begin with our affirmations.

[30 seconds]

This meditation is designed to bring positive changes in your health and fitness. Real change begins in the mind with the change in our thought process. Therefore, we will combine mediation with affirmations and positive statements. They can reprogram the mind by replacing the negative thinking created by the bad habits.

We will repeat each affirmation thrice. When saying the affirmation the first time, we will feel it sinking deep into our mind. On the second time, we will feel the meditation sinking deep into our body. And on the third time, we feel the positive change sinking into our soul.

So let's begin

First say these affirmations for your body. "I am confident in my body. I am confident about my body. As I bring positive changes in my lifestyle, my body responds positively. I nourish my body with healthy wholesome and fresh food. I make healthy food choices that aid my weight loss journey. Everything works out to my highest benefit."

[5 seconds]

Now repeat these affirmations for your mind. "I am confident in my body. I am confident about my body. As I bring positive changes in my lifestyle, my body responds positively. I nourish my body with healthy wholesome and fresh food. I make healthy food choices that aid my weight loss journey. Everything works out to my highest benefit."

[5 seconds]

Now let these affirmations sink deep into your soul. "I am confident in my body. I am confident about my body. As I bring positive changes in my lifestyle, my body responds positively. I nourish my body with healthy wholesome and fresh food. I make healthy food choices that aid my weight loss journey. Everything works out to my highest benefit."

[10 seconds]

First say these affirmations for your body. "I realise that physical change follows mental change. I gradually move towards the best version of my physical body in terms of weight and size. Change is coming naturally and effortlessly and I am completely enjoying the process of body loss. I have all that it takes to achieve my ideal body weight. Weight loss is as natural for me as breathing in and breathing out. I am all in for a positive body transformation."

[5 seconds]

Now repeat these affirmations for your mind. "I realise that physical change follows mental change. I gradually move towards the best version of my physical body in terms of weight and size. Change is coming naturally and effortlessly and I am completely enjoying the process of body loss. I have all that it takes to achieve my ideal body weight. Weight loss is as natural for me as breathing in and breathing out. I am all in for a positive body transformation."

[5 seconds]

Now let these affirmations sink deep into your soul. "I realise that physical change follows mental change. I gradually move towards the best version of my physical body in terms of weight and size. Change is coming naturally and effortlessly and I am completely enjoying the process of body loss. I have all that it takes to achieve my ideal body weight. Weight loss is as natural for me as breathing in and breathing out. I am all in for a positive body transformation."

[10 seconds]

First say these affirmations for your body. "I eat to nourish my body. I desire foods that support my healthy body. I enjoy low calorie food. I have fast metabolism. I am motivated to achieve my weight loss goals. I am getting rid of all the extra and unwanted fat from my body"

[5 seconds]

Now repeat these affirmations for your mind. "I eat to nourish my body. I desire foods that support my healthy body. I enjoy low calorie food. I have fast metabolism. I am motivated to achieve my weight loss goals. I am getting rid of all the extra and unwanted fat from my body"

[5 seconds]

Now let these affirmations sink deep into your soul. "I eat to nourish my body. I desire foods that support my healthy body. I enjoy low calorie food. I have fast metabolism. I am motivated to achieve my weight loss goals. I am getting rid of all the extra and unwanted fat from my body"

[10 seconds]

First say these affirmations for your body.

"I eat mindfully and consciously. I eat only what I need. I enjoy eating more fruits and vegetables. I find healthy ways to comfort myself. I eat natural foods. I am open to a new way of eating. I am absorbing all the good nutrients and nourishment from the food I eat."

[5 seconds]

Now repeat these affirmations for your mind. "I eat mindfully and consciously. I eat only what I need. I enjoy eating more fruits and vegetables. I find healthy ways to comfort myself. I eat natural foods. I am open to a new way of eating. I am absorbing all the good nutrients and nourishment from the food I eat."

[5 seconds]

Now let these affirmations sink deep into your soul. "I eat mindfully and consciously. I eat only what I need. I enjoy eating more fruits and vegetables. I find healthy ways to comfort myself. I eat natural foods. I am open to a new way of eating. I am absorbing all the good nutrients and nourishment from the food I eat."

[10 seconds]

First say these affirmations for your body. "My health is perfect in many ways. I am getting stronger and slimmer every day. I enjoy of variety of wholesome food. I am in control of what I eat. I crave whole foods and healthy foods. Healthy food is working wonders for my body as I become fitter, slimmer, and healthier."

[5 seconds]

Now repeat these affirmations for your mind. "My health is perfect in many ways. I am getting stronger and slimmer every day. I enjoy of variety of wholesome food. I am in control of what I eat. I crave whole foods and healthy foods. Healthy food is working wonders for my body as I become fitter, slimmer, and healthier."

[5 seconds]

Now let these affirmations sink deep into your soul. "My health is perfect in many ways. I am getting stronger and slimmer every day. I enjoy of variety of wholesome food. I am in control of what I eat. I crave whole foods and healthy foods. Healthy food is working wonders for my body as I become fitter, slimmer, and healthier."

[10 seconds]

First say these affirmations for your body. "I am filled with enthusiasm and energy. I love to exercise in a way that is fun to me. I am getting lighter and lean. I enjoy my workout sessions. I love how exercise makes my body and mind feel. I am at the peak of my health and fitness and am maintaining that perfect state of being."

[5 seconds]

Now repeat these affirmations for your mind. "I am filled with enthusiasm and energy. I love to exercise in a way that is fun to me. I am getting lighter and lean. I enjoy my workout sessions. I love how exercise makes my body and mind feel. I am at the peak of my health and fitness and am maintaining that perfect state of being."

[5 seconds]

Now let these affirmations sink deep into your soul. "I am filled with enthusiasm and energy. I love to exercise in a way that is fun to me. I am getting lighter and lean. I enjoy my workout sessions. I love how exercise makes my body and mind feel. I am at the peak of my health and fitness and am maintaining that perfect state of being."

[10 seconds]

First say these affirmations for your body. "I choose to drink lot of water and stay healthy. I love to find fun ways to exercise in regular basis. I am in control of my weight. Weight loss is happening naturally and organically. I am getting closer and closer every day to my perfect body."

[5 seconds]

Now repeat these affirmations for your mind. "I choose to drink lot of water and stay healthy. I love to find fun ways to exercise in regular basis. I am in control of my weight. Weight loss is happening naturally and organically. I am getting closer and closer every day to my perfect body."

[5 seconds]

Now let these affirmations sink deep into your soul. "I choose to drink lot of water and stay healthy. I love to find fun ways to exercise in regular basis. I am in control of my weight. Weight loss is happening naturally and organically. I am getting closer and closer every day to my perfect body."

[10 seconds]

First say these affirmations for your body. "I am in control of my emotions. I know when to say no to food. I can differentiate physical hunger from emotional hunger and will eat only when I am physically hungry. My wise eating choices are showing marvellous results. I am grateful for having this body that is capable for effectively losing weight."

[5 seconds]

Now repeat these affirmations for your mind. "I am in control of my emotions. I know when to say no to food. I can differentiate physical hunger from emotional hunger and will eat only when I am physically hungry. My wise eating choices are showing marvellous results. I am grateful for having this body that is capable for effectively losing weight."

[5 seconds]

Now let these affirmations sink deep into your soul. "I am in control of my emotions. I know when to say no to food. I can differentiate physical hunger from emotional hunger and will eat only when I am physically hungry. My wise eating choices are showing marvellous results. I am grateful for having this body that is capable for effectively losing weight."

[10 seconds]

First say these affirmations for your body. "I release the past and let it go. I am healthy and happy. I trust myself fully. I am grateful for my health. I am kind to myself. My body is shedding the burdens of my past."

[5 seconds]

Now repeat these affirmations for your mind. "I release the past and let it go. I am healthy and happy. I trust myself fully. I am grateful for my health. I am kind to myself. My body is shedding the burdens of my past."

[5 seconds]

Now let these affirmations sink deep into your soul. "I release the past and let it go. I am healthy and happy. I trust myself fully. I am grateful for my health. I am kind to myself. My body is shedding the burdens of my past."

[10 seconds]

First say these affirmations for your body. "I am getting lighter and stronger every day. I enjoy taking good care of myself. I can do anything I set my mind to. My actions and behaviour support my perfect weight. I am excited about a new way of being lighter, fitter, and healthier. I embrace a life full of limitless possibilities"

[5 seconds]

Now repeat these affirmations for your mind. "I am getting lighter and stronger every day. I enjoy taking good care of myself. I can do anything I set my mind to. My actions and behaviour support my perfect weight. I am excited about a new way of being lighter, fitter, and healthier. I embrace a life full of limitless possibilities"

[5 seconds]

Now let these affirmations sink deep into your soul. "I am getting lighter and stronger every day. I enjoy taking good care of myself. I can do anything I set my mind to. My actions and behaviour support my perfect weight. I am excited about a new way of being lighter, fitter, and healthier. I embrace a life full of limitless possibilities"

[10 seconds]

First say these affirmations for your body. "I know deep within me that a big positive change is around the corner. I am ready and prepared to lead a fully transformed life. Everything in my life is turning in my favour for a healthy, fit, slim and a more attractive version of me. I am a new person without the burdens of my past. Life is full of sunshine and positivity. I am on my way to my physical, mental, and spiritual best."

[5 seconds]

Now repeat these affirmations for your mind. "I know deep within me that a big positive change is around the corner. I am ready and prepared to lead a fully transformed life. Everything in my life is turning in my favour for a healthy, fit, slim and a more attractive version of me. I am a new person without the burdens of my past. Life is full of sunshine and positivity. I am on my way to my physical, mental, and spiritual best."

[5 seconds]

Now let these affirmations sink deep into your soul. "I know deep within me that a big positive change is around the corner. I am ready and prepared to lead a fully transformed life. Everything in my life is turning in my favour for a healthy, fit, slim and a more attractive version of me. I am a new person without the burdens of my past. Life is full of sunshine and positivity. I am on my way to my physical, mental, and spiritual best."

10. Ideal Weight hypnosis – 30 minutes

Lie down in a comfortable position. Relax your shoulders, your head and your neck.

[5 seconds]

When you are ready just breathe. Breathe deep down into diaphragm, just notice the actual raise and fall.

[5 seconds]

Breathing in a wonderful relaxation and calm and peace. Breathing out every tension, just relaxing and releasing them.

[5 seconds]

Becoming aware of natural flow of air to in and out of your nostrils.

[5 seconds]

Don't force your breath let it find its own natural rhythm. Just gently let them be.

[5 seconds]

And then bring your awareness to the crown of your head. Become aware of how tight your scalp is. Consciously let those muscles relax and as you do so, feel the tension sliding of the top. Relax. Relax. Relax.

[5 seconds]

Breathing into it and just releasing and letting it go. Bring your focus down to your forehead. Relax. Relax. Relax. And as you consciously release each and one all of those muscles, just notice how wide and how smooth is your forehead is. Just release and let it go. Relax. Relax. Relax.

[5 seconds]

Bring focus all the muscles around your eyes. Your eyes that work so hard. And as you release the tension from your eyes, they feel so relaxed. They had been working hard all day. And now they have finally got the time to relax. So just let them relax. Relax. Relax. Relax.

[5 seconds]

Become aware of your cheek bones and just let them relax. Relax. Relax. Relax. Let the tension just drift away.

[5 seconds]

Drop your jaw to allow a bit of space in between your taste.

[5 seconds]

And now bring your focus to your tongue. As you bring that focus to your tongue become aware of how heavy that feels. If you just allow it to fall to your mouth. It's getting heavier and heavier. So, now just relax and breathe. Relax. Relax. Relax. Breathing in and just releasing any tension, just let them go.

[5 seconds]

Relax your muscles around your lips and your chin.

[5 seconds]

Follow your jaw line around to the back of your neck.

[5 seconds]

And then the muscles around the top of your spine, one by one just let them relax down through your neck. One by one consciously just letting them go. And just relax and breathe.

[5 seconds]

Take a deep breath in and just relax and let go.

[5 seconds]

Bring your awareness down to your shoulders. And first of all just lift them slightly and then drop them down and just let them relax and let all tension go. Punch them back up to your back and then just let them go. Let them relax and breathe.

[5 seconds]

All of your focus to your left hand shoulder. Become aware of every muscle and as you do consciously, let each those muscles relax. All through your shoulder blades feel your shoulder dropping down and as you do feel the tension melt away. Breathe down into your shoulder and release every bit of tension.

[5 seconds]

Follow that relaxation down into your left bicep and just let that relax.

[5 seconds]

Down into your left elbow and just relax that elbow down.

[5 seconds]

Your left forearm, relax that left wrist and manage your focus to your left hand, consciously relax all of the muscle.

[5 seconds]

And follow it through the each fingertip. Your thumb, your first finger, your middle finger, your third finger, your little finger. With every muscle be in relax breath down into the arm, releasing every piece of tension and just relax and breathe.

[5 seconds]

Now bring your attention to right hand shoulder. And again focus on all the muscles. And one by one allow them to relax. And as you do notice how it feels, notice how that feels to relax the muscles allow the tension just melt away. Take a deep breath in and down into the shoulder and just release and let it go and relax.

[5 seconds]

Follow down into your right hand bicep and just relax and breathe that right elbow and relax your right forearm, right wrist, and all the muscles in your right hand.

[5 seconds]

Follow it through your tip of right thumb, your right first finger, middle finger, third finger and little finger. Breathe down right away through your entire arm, just release and let it go. And relax and breathe.

[5 seconds]

Bring your attention to the front of your neck and throat. And just let the muscles around that area to relax. Follow down into your chest and let each of those muscles relax as you do feel the tension lifting off. Breathe down into that area and just relax and breathe.

[5 seconds]

Working down behind your rib cage. And your mid rift .feel the sides of your body to just relaxing , your stomach muscles, and just everything release. Release and let it go.

[5 seconds]

Bring your focus to your spine, work away down each and every muscle. Follow it through the sides of your body and across your entire back. Just relax and breathe.

[5 seconds]

Get in to the center of your back slowly but surely touching each and every one of those muscles with your fingers one by one. Releasing tension by tension and relaxing muscle by muscle. All the way across to the edges. And just relax and breathe as you get to the bottom of your spine.

[5 seconds]

Just follow this relaxation down into your hips. Let the tension just melt away as all the muscles in your hips really start to relax. Just feel the melt into whatever is beneath. And just release the let everything go. Relax. Relax. Relax. Take a deep breath in and just allow that flow through every particle of your back and your torso and through your hips. Just relax and breathe.

[5 seconds]

Put all of your focus on your right end thigh and consciously all the muscle relax. And follow that relaxation to your right knee and calves. Relax your right ankle, and release every muscle on your feet. Go through your hips to each of your toes. 1, 2, 3, 4, and 5. Now breathe.

[5 seconds]

Bring your attention to your left end thigh. And release each of those muscles. And let it all go. Relax that left knee, follow that release in to your calves, your left ankle, your left foot, and to your toes. 1, 2, 3, 4 and 5.

[5 seconds]

Breathe in and let it just flow from the crown of your head all the way through every part of your head, neck, torso, your limbs, feet ,into the tip of both toes and just relax and breathe.

[5 seconds]

Scan your body from your crown, all the way to your toes and back up to your crown. And any way you still feel any tension. Put all of your focus on that area. And consciously allow those muscles to just completely release and let everything go.

[5 seconds]

Bring your focus back to your breathing.

[1 minute]

In your third eye, I want you to imagine your body at its ideal weight.

[5 seconds]

Your body looks perfect. You feel healthier and so good about yourself. Notice how perfect your body looks now. You have always wanted to look this way. Now you can feel that emotion. Notice the confidence as you walk. You feel so confident, so much alive. You have never so confident before. You feel so good not only because of the way you look but also from the inside. You know that you are beautiful, dashing person from the inside as well as from the outside. And with head held high, you walk. You walk with full confidence. Imagine yourself as vividly as possible. Visualize the healthy, slim, fit, attractive you. This is who you truly are. Hold this image of your true nature in your third eye for a while.

[10 seconds]

And as you hold on to this image in your mind, only positive thoughts come to your mind. You know you are a positive soul that deserves the best of everything. You deserve to look good. You deserve to feel good. And that fit, healthy, smart version of you is a complete possibility. You just need to make a few good choices. We may not be in control of what happens to us but we have full control over how we react. You need not be controlled by your emotions. You are the master of your emotions. You are the master of your body. And you can make good, healthy decisions to become the healthier version of you. Healthy choices transform you in a positive way. They transform not only your physical self but also how you feel about yourself. They make you feel confident and competent. You see yourself as an individual who can achieve anything. Because when you can control your mind and make good choices when it comes to what you eat, you can use that mental strength to make good choices on other aspects of your life as well. And you will be full of unshakeable confidence within you. And once you reach that level of mindset, making healthy food choices no longer seems like a difficulty or a compulsion, it becomes a natural act. Then you look for healthy food no matter where you are. Unhealthy, fatty food will repulse you.

[5 seconds]

Now you understand that it's all about your mindset. Picture again now, you are thinner, leaner and healthier you. Notice how you look, notice how your muscles are lean and firm and how your skin is tight and glowing. You have never felt so good before. Notice how comfortable you are in your cloths. Notice how gracefully you walk and jog and run and exercise. Isn't that amazing? Notice how you move about, how you dance and how you play and go about your day doing all the physical activities so gracefully. Everybody around you just can't take their eyes off you.

[5 seconds]

You slip into your cloths perfectly. And whatever you wear, it looks so good on you. As if the cloth, the material were meant just for you. And you dress and move so confidently.

Feel that confidence. Feel yourself walk with that confidence. Feel how well it feels to look and be so healthy, so fit, so slim, so active and so attractive. You have never felt so confident before. Feel how wonderful it is to be to have that perfect body. Feel the feeling.

[5 seconds]

Now float into that perfect body of yours. How does it feel? You have a mirror in front of you, look into that mirror. How do you look? How do you feel in your new perfect-looking body? It sure feels so good.

[5 seconds]

This is your body. This is how you would be looking. Your subconscious mind has received the message. From now on, it will look for ways to make you go forward on the path of looking this way. It will make you stay away from all the unhealthy food that corrupts your health and well being. So, for now you just rest and relax and fall into a deep slumber. The message has been received. It has been received well. From now on, you have to make wise choices for food and exercise. Don't worry about the resources and the strength, the universe will provide for all the requirements. You subconscious mind know how to react. So, just stay on the right path of diet. You will keep meeting people who will nudge you on the right path. You will get the right advice at the right time but you need to act on them. The subconscious mind has received the message and has already starting working on how to make you turn into the healthier, fitter and more attractive version of you.

11. Taming Addictions – 40 minutes

Hi, welcome to this special meditation. Just sit in any comfortable position. Do not be very casual. Your entire focus should be on this meditation. At the same time you have the liberty to sit in a position of your choice that is relaxing and keeps you alert as well.

So, beginning with bringing the awareness to the now – the precious present moment.

[5 seconds]

Now, take a deep breath in. Inhaling through the nose. And release. Exhaling through the mouth.

Very good.

Now another deep breath in through the nose. And out through the mouth.

Notice how relaxed you feel after each breath.

And another deep breath in through the nose. And out through the mouth.

And feeling relaxed.

And three more deep breaths at your own intensity. Going as deep as you can with the inhalation through the nose. And releasing with an open mouth.

[10 seconds]

And relax. Feeling so calm, so peaceful.

Today, we are going to work on your food cravings. We all enjoy food, don't we. But sometimes we tend to indulge too much. And then we later regret that act of overeating.

So, if you are sort of addicted to certain kind of food or food in general, this meditation is for you. Even if you are not addicted, but wish to control your cravings for certain food, maybe your favourite burger or pizza or of you are fond of sweet, anything you feel you can't stop yourself from eating and then overeating, this meditation will help.

Meditations are not about some random visualisations. They strike where the problem exists. So, when we talk about cravings or addictions, they are basically associated with your lower three chakras or energy centres of your body.

So, through this meditation, we will try to balance your basic chakras. And when they begin to balance and align, you will notice a higher level of control and balance within you. So, let the change happen organically.

So, beginning with bringing your awareness to your physical body. Notice how you feel right now.

[5 seconds]

Maintain a gentle focus on your breathing. The inflow and the outflow of air.

[10 seconds]

Now, at the base of your spine, just where your back touches the surface beneath when you sit, at that point, I want you to imagine a red coloured ball. This is the seat of your Root Chakra, the first of the seven chakras in your body. Coloured in red, the Root Chakra governs your basic needs, your survival instincts. When your Root Chakra is imbalanced, you feel insecure or may indulge in hoarding. You may eat more than you want to because you are insecure. You are afraid to postpone the act of eating. You want everything now. You are afraid, you are insecure; hence you eat more. And then you gain weight. So, we need to balance this chakra of survival and security.

Now, visualise your Root Chakra as a red colour ball at the base of your spine.

And from the base of your spine, visualise roots – like roots of a big tree – growing and entering the Earth beneath you. Visualise the roots growing and multiplying and spreading. The roots are going deeper and deeper into the Earth and they are spreading far away as well. So, these roots are growing vertically as well as horizontally and spreading across the surface of the Earth.

[5 seconds]

Now visualise that the roots have reached the centre of the Earth and have stabilised there. Create a mental image of this scene. You sitting still, with roots growing from your tailbone and spreading deep into the Earth and connecting you with the Earth's centre.

[5 seconds]

I want you to feel the connection deep within you. The connection, the bond with the mother Earth. Feel it deep within you.

[5 seconds]

Feel the protection that the Mother Earth provides. You are safe, you are secure in her protective embrace.

[5 seconds]

Mother Earth takes care of you. She has always been taking care of you. She nurtures you, nourishes you, supports you. You need not worry for anything under her protection, under her watch.

[5 seconds]

Feel the support, the security, the strength that comes with this association.

[10 seconds]

Now bring your focus again at the base of your spine. Visualising your Root Chakra as a red coloured ball. And visualise this ball spinning at its seat. Spinning in clockwise direction. And it spins faster and faster. And as it swirls and generates momentum, you can feel all your cravings, all your insecurities, all your fears and addictions being released from different parts of your body. And visualise these addictions and cravings as black coloured smoke flowing towards the Red coloured ball of energy swirling at the base of your spine.

All your insecurities and fears and traumas, or any weakness that you think that you have, visualise them as black coloured smoke moving towards and collecting at your Root Chakra.

[5 seconds]

Visualise this for all your addictions and cravings one by one. Collect all your unwanted habits and negativity at your red coloured Root Chakra.

[2 minutes]

Now, you have collected all your cravings as black coloured smoke in your Root Chakra, the chakra of stability and security. I want you to visualise that you are transferring all the black coloured negativity from your tailbone into the Earth through the roots that reach the centre of the Earth.

Visualise the black coloured negativity travelling down the roots and being released in the Earth. The mother Earth is accepting all your negativity. The mother Earth is accepting all your cravings and addictions.

[5 seconds]

And as you release your cravings and insecurities and transfer them to Mother Earth, feel a sense of relief. Feel as if you are releasing all your stress and all your worries. Feel free. Feel light. Keep releasing your negativity. Mother Earth will embrace all.

[20 seconds]

Release all your black coloured negativity until you become empty. Feel as if there is nothing negative inside of you. There is nothing that controls you. Feel light. Feel free.

[10 seconds]

Feel as if the Mother Earth is whispering in your ears, "Don't worry. I have your back. No matter how many times you fall, I will be there. I will always be there to support you. I will always be there to protect you. You are safe. You are protected. Whenever you will the craving, don't just give up. You know you have to the strength to withstand any type of craving or addiction. Remind yourself of this connection. And whenever you ask for my help, I will be there. I will send you my positive energies as I am sending you right now."

[5 seconds]

And now from these roots that are the loving embrace Mother Earth, feel bright white positive light of healing entering your body through the base of your spine, energising your red coloured Root Chakra, and then visualise this white healing light spreading all across your body and reinvigorating all your organs and each and every cell of your body.

[5 seconds]

Feel every part of your body being filled with this positive energy that the Mother Earth has sent for you. This energy will help you fight any pangs of hunger or cravings that you might face any time in the future.

[5 seconds]

Feel this positive energy in every cell, every organ of your body. Thank the Mother Earth for sending this positive, healing light.

[1 minute]

Now, we are going to work on your second chakra, the Sacral Chakra, which is associated with pleasures. So, when we indulge in cravings and food addictions it is mainly because we seek pleasures for our sense of taste. It is also associated with our ability to adapt to changes, our intimacy, self-gratification, and how we identify with our feelings. At the level of energies, it is basically because of an imbalance in our Sacral Chakra. This chakra is located just below your navel and is of orange colour.

[5 seconds]

Now, I want you to visualise yourself standing in front of a pond in the middle of forest. It's a full moon night and you can see the image of the moon in the clear water of the pond. Water is a representation of your Sacral Chakra and your emotional depths. Tip your toe in feel the water on your skin. It's just the perfect temperature – so soothing and so peaceful. Step into the pond and keep going in till you are shoulder deep in the water. Feel a sense of relief and relaxation, as if the water is taking away all your stress and worries.

[5 seconds]

Feel the pleasure of the clean, soothing water against your skin.

[5 seconds]

Now, I want you to take a dip and submerse yourself into the water. And as you are inside the water, you feel that as if your arms and legs have been chained and you can't move. You use all your force but the chains are too strong. And then suddenly a bright light comes from above breaks all the chains, one by one, setting you free. And as you release these chains, feel yourself letting go of all your food addictions and cravings.

One by one, free yourself of these chains, free yourself all the cravings and addictions.

[10 seconds]

And as you set yourself free, you rise up to the surface of water, you notice it's dawn and the sun is rising across the horizon. It's a new day, it's a new beginning of your life. And you feel free and light.

[1 minute]

Now, we will be focusing on your third chakra, solar plexus. It is associated with your willpower, your discipline and your sense of self. An imbalance in this chakra weakens your control over your actions and you tend to give up too easily on your diet and exercise goals. Now, we are going to balance your Solar Plexus Chakra, located between your navel and lower ribs. It is associated with colour yellow and element fire.

[5 seconds]

Now, I want you to visualise yourself standing in front of a roaring bonfire. Even though you are at a considerable distance, you can still feel the heat of the flames on your skin.

[5 seconds]

You get an intuition that you need to walk through this bonfire. After a little hesitancy, you decide to walk through the flames and begin to march towards it. And as you step into the fire, the flames turn a brilliant healing white and you stand in your power allowing the fire to burn away your addictions, your self-doubt, your limiting beliefs, low self-esteem, any old stories you tell yourself about why you can't lose weight. The flames burn them all away. Your power has been unleashed. You step out of the flame. You have been reborn. The new you is free of addictions, cravings. The new you has the discipline and self control.

[5 seconds]

Now for the next few minutes I want you to focus on your three chakras, the red coloured Root Chakra located at the base of your spine, the orange coloured Sacral Chakra, located just below your navel, and the yellow coloured Solar Plexus located between your navel and lower ribs.

[5 seconds]

Feel them rotating in spinning on their axis in clockwise direction and in full alignment with one another.

Charge them with the following intentions:

"I let go of all my past habits that no longer serve my health and hygiene. My mind, body, and energies are in perfect harmony. I am getting closer and closer every day to my Perfect body"

[5 seconds]

"I let go of all my past habits that no longer serve my health and hygiene. My mind, body, and energies are in perfect harmony. I am getting closer and closer every day to my Perfect body"

[5 seconds]

"I let go of all my past habits that no longer serve my health and hygiene. My mind, body, and energies are in perfect harmony. I am getting closer and closer every day to my Perfect body"

[10 seconds]

Now, bring your awareness back to your physical body. Join your palms at your chest centre in the Namaste position. Thank the energies. Thank your chakras. Gently rub your palms against each other.

Bring your palms to your eyes, gently massaging them. And when you are ready, come back.

12. Journey to your ideal weight – 60 minutes

Lie down in a comfortable position. You may choose to close your eyes or keep it open. You may resume your day after the meditation ends or you may choose to go to sleep. Take your time to adjust your body for a relaxing experience.

[5 seconds]

We will begin by bringing the awareness to the physical body. Recognize the space you are in.

[5 seconds]

Be aware of your body, your presence. Now gently bring your focus your feet. Notice the sensations in your feet, just notice without judgment. Do you sense anything?

[5 seconds]

Allow your toes to wiggle. Allow your ankles to roll. Relax your body.

[5 seconds]

Imagine as if you are sending your breath down to your feet as if the breath is travelling through your nose down to the lungs and through the abdomen all the way down to your feet. Let your focus rest with your feet this way for a few more moments. If your mind wanders away, gently bring your focus back to your feet.

[5 seconds]

Now, your gently bring your focus to your legs. To your calves and kneesyou're your thighs. You might feel the touch of clothing or blanket or you may feel nothing at all. Feel the sensation to your experiencing throughout your legs. Do you feel any sensations?

[5 seconds]

Breathe into and breathe out of your legs. If you find an area of discomfort, just acknowledge it and allow it to pass without changing it. Breathe into your legs, allow the legs to dissolve in your mind. When you focus on a body part, feel it letting go of any stress it may be holding onto.

[5 seconds]

Send your breath now to your pelvis and lower back. When you focus on a body part, feel it letting go of any stress it may be holding onto. Softening and releasing and relaxing as you breathe in and out.

[5 seconds]

Now, I want you to turn your focus to the abdomen and then your chest. Notice the physical sensations, such as breathing and internal feelings like hunger or fullness. With each breath let go of tension you are carrying. When you focus on a body part, feel it letting go of any stress it may be holding onto. If you notice opinion or judgments of any type forming above these areas, gently release them. And try to notice any sensations. Do you feel anything?

[5 seconds]

Feel your clothing, feel the process of digestion with the belly gently rising and falling with each breath.

[5 seconds]

Now on the next breath, gently bring your focus to your hands and finger tips. Breathing in to out of this area as if your hands are doing the breathing.

[5 seconds]

If your thoughts wander, gently bring it back to the sensation of your hands. When you focus on a body part, feel it letting go of any stress it may be holding onto. Allow your focus to go up into your arms. As you exhale you may experience the softening and releasing gently. Continue to breathe.

[5 seconds]

Send your focus now to your neck region, your shoulders and the front area. This is a spot where we often have some stress lurking. Be with the sensations here. Feel it. It could be tightness or the sensation of holding on. When you focus on a body part, feel it letting go of any stress it may be holding onto. Let go of any thoughts or stories you are telling about this area. As you breathe feel the tension rolling off your shoulders. When you focus on a body part, feel it letting go of any stress it may be holding onto.

[5 seconds]

Bring your focus to your face and head. Notice the moment of the air as you breathe in to or out of the nostrils and mouth.

[5 seconds]

As you exhale notice the softening of any tension you may be holding. Now, I want you to allow your focus to expand out to the body as a whole. Bring in to your awareness up of your head, down to the soles of your feet. Feel the gentle rhythm of the breath as it moves through the body.

[30 seconds]

You are practicing this hypnosis meditation so that you can reach your goal of being at your ideal weight. So that you can lose weight in an easy and healthy way and in a way that is just right for you, your body and your health. And you have wanted to do this, sometimes so you know exactly what it is, and exactly that you want. So just remind your subconscious mind just what you already want. Your subconscious mind knows exactly what weight you want to be. It knows exactly what size you want to be. And it knows exactly how you want to feel. It also knows how you want to look and also why you want to be this weight. And why you want to feel this way. Why you want to look this way. It knows exactly what will this mean to you. And your subconscious mind knows how reaching your goal will change your life.

Your subconscious mind knows and understands everything. It knows how this exercise will benefit your health and wellbeing. It knows very well that consciously and subconsciously it is appropriate and beneficial to lose that extra weight. This is your conscious decision and your own desire to lose that extra weight. And if your mind wanders, let it be, and if you feel sleepy, don't force yourself to stay awake because your subconscious mind is listening. And I want you to know that no matter how difficult it may seem, but when your subconscious mind is commanded, you will find it so easy to lose weight. From now on, never again you are going to eat unless you feel the physiological hunger. Not just that, from now on, you will only eat those foods that are good for your body. Your cravings will make a one eighty degree flip and from now on you will only consume those foods that are good for your body. It is better to consume something you are delighted with.

[5 seconds]

You will find that when you are hungry, you are just craving for foods and products that are good for your fitness and you find yourself turning away from any food or drink that would have harmed your physical body in the past. You will always sit down to eat when you are physiologically hungry, and when you sit down to eat you will chew every bite very slowly. You will chew every bite almost twenty times so that your food is almost liquid by the time you swallow it. And you will realise that this makes it so much easier for your body to take all the good nutrients from the food that you just consumed. And you receive proper nourishment form your food.

[5 seconds]

And your subconscious mind knows how important water is for your health. So, from now on, you will enjoy drinking water more than ever before. And you will soon find yourself taking in more and more water. You will enjoy the cleansing properties of the water. You enjoy the feel of the wonderful water going down your throat. You can feel it recharging you and refreshing you and cleansing every cell of your being. You can imagine it brightening your skin and your eyes. You like the lovely taste of the water. And you are drinking more and more water than ever. You are drinking much more water than you normally do. And this is working wonders or you.

[5 seconds]

You will notice that this healthy diet and water consumption is doing wanders for you. You are beginning to lose weight. Not just that, your stomach is getting smaller and smaller till it is the size that you believe is perfect for you. With every day that passes, you notice that naturally you will want to consume smaller and smaller quantities of food. Your appetite is getting smaller. And you feel that you have eaten enough after consuming a small quantity of food.

[5 seconds]

You will remember that the heavy feeling of having eaten too much and you will never want to have that stuffed feeling ever again. You visualize your stomach as a small vessel. And from now on, when you eat food, your brain will receive the signal that your stomach is full a lot quicker than usual. And, quite obviously, you will be chewing every bite very, very slowly, which will also help your brain in receiving that signal that you are now satiated and that it is time for you to stop eating. And it is not just about eating slowly but enjoying every bite. Every bite that goes into your bite, it fills your mouth with different flavours. And you savour every flavour. You will be amazed by how much good your taste buds feel, how much work they do, and how much wonderful feelings of different tastes they offer you. You have never felt that food could be so tasty. Earlier you used to eat unmindfully. Your mind used to wander every time you ate food. But from now, you will be present in every moment of your meals. You will be fully conscious when you eat. and you will enjoy the food so much more. You will notice and enjoy the different flavours and textures of the food you eat and you will chew your food properly, about twenty times. And when you eat mindfully, you won't reach for the unnecessary things and you won't seek to finish everything that's on your plate if you are full. You find it very easy to put down the knife and fork and say to yourself, "I have had enough. That's the perfect amount for me. I feel satiated." And you say it again, "I have had enough. That's the perfect amount for me. I feel satiated." And one more time, "I have had enough. That's the perfect amount for me. I feel satiated." Your subconscious mind is absorbing these positive affirmations.

[5 seconds]

You can either consume the left over on the plate another time or you can throw them away. Either way it is far better than consuming them now. It is always better than to keep eating when it's not required to do so. It's best to stop when your body has signalled you that it's got all it needs now. So, from now on, you listen to your body. It is as if you are sync with your body. With each day this synchronicity increases. And it is working wonders for you. And you are giving your body all it needs and exactly how much it needs. Not a bite more, not a bite less. No more than that is necessary for your body. You are feeding your body with all the nice and healthy food. And you don't want to feed anything to your body that isn't nice.

[5 seconds]

From now on, you are enjoying a new and novel way of eating. You now eat your food very, very slowly. And it's not just about the speed. It's about eating mindfully. You put down your cutlery on the dining table between the bites. And you eat mindfully, completely enjoying the food which is in your mouth. You are in no hurry. And because you enjoy and think only about bite that is in your mouth, it will taste much better now. You become so mindful and so much sensitive to the taste and smells of whatever it is that you are eating. From now on, you are far more satisfied and happy with every meal that you consume. And this is because you are in sync with the tastes, with the smells, the senses, and textures, more in sync than you were ever before. The food tastes amazingly well. You eat not just slowly but mindfully. From now on, you notice that you consume much less but are fully satiated with whatever small amount you eat. you take in all the nutrients and nourishment. Your body is responding beautifully to all the changes you are making to your eating habits. And you are always enjoying your food. And if your mind wanders, let it be, and if you feel sleepy, don't force yourself to stay awake because your subconscious mind is listening.

[5 seconds]

From now on, you will never have any feeling of guilt or anxiety about any meal or whether it's going to increase your weight. From now on, you will look forward to preparing food and you will look forward to eating it not just to fill your tummy but because it's a new experience altogether. You enjoy everything about your food and you find it very easy to stop as soon as you are satiated. You are fully aware that you can eat it again or may be the next time.

[5 seconds]

From now on, any foods that are unhealthy and bad for you, such as sweets, oily foods, snacks generate feelings of repulsion within you. And because these unhealthy foods are repulsive to you, you will now lose that weight very easily and effortlessly. You will notice that with each passing day, your body will change for the better and it will keep changing until you reach your target of your ideal weight that you want to be. And when you reach the ideal weight you want to be, you will notice that your weight then becomes nearly constant. And you will remain at your ideal weight and you will continue to consume in this healthy way. And not just that, you will find it so easy to maintain this healthy lifestyle. And also, you will so good and so joyful. You will find yourself being more energetic and active. And you will feel your mindset transforming for the better. You will find exercising very interesting. And exercising can be in any for you like, including jogging, swimming, or playing an outdoor sport. From now on, you will find that you can effortlessly exercise more and it gives wonderful results. And the more you exercise the more energetic you feel. And the better you feel, the more you want to do your exercise. The more you want to move your body and you really want to. It becomes another healthy thing that you really look forward to do. It feels Easy and effortless and brings so much happiness to your life. And you feel so good about your life in every way imaginable. From now on, you Find it so easy to maintain these healthy eating habits. And not just that, you find it so exciting to go out and exercise because you really want to do so. Because from now on, you really enjoy the physical activities that keep you fit and it good shape. You notice that people are now complementing you so much. They are often saying to you that you are looking so much better. And it is not about the complements. The thing is that now you are feeling so much better about your body and the way you look. You fitting perfectly in your favourite cloths that you always wanted to wear. And it is as if the unwanted weight is melting away. And you are feeling so good about everything. And a wonderful thing is that these beautiful feelings are going to grow and they are going to multiply. And now, you are so are so much more excited about the future. There is optimism in you. You are thinking in your head, "How fit am I going to look this time next week. How much better am I going feel in the coming days?" And there is so much confidence in you now that you are now unstoppable. This wonderful feeling will carry on and on and on. And you notice that your mind is full of ideas about what you going to do next. You know everything will be good now, and everything will turn in your favour. And you begin to feel good about yourself. You will walk with so much more confidence. You will talk with so much more confidence. And you will think and act with full confidence. Your subconscious mind has received the commands. It is already working on them. All you need to do is relax and enter the deeper levels of hypnosis.

I want you to know that you have every right to enjoy a healthy and fit body. You have so much respect for your mind, your health and your body. And you know how want to look, how you want to feel. And that's why you have chosen your ideal weight and your ideal size. And from now on, anytime you think about yourself, you will see your ideal size and your ideal weight. Because from now on, that is the real you that is in making. And so you will from now on visualize the real you. Every single part of you, every cell in your body understands now your great desire to get to and maintain this ideal weight and size for you.

And if your mind wanders, let it be, and if you feel sleepy, don't force yourself to stay awake because your subconscious mind is listening.

[5 seconds]

Now, I want you to imagine that you are in your own safe place, a very peaceful place. And you feel slim, healthy, and attractive. Here, you are enjoying being the real you. And now visualise that in front of you there is a beautiful mirror. And in that mirror you see yourself smiling so wide. You have never seen yourself be so happy. You are amazed at what you see in the mirror. You are just your perfect weight and size. You turn around and see yourself from different angles, and from every angle you look just perfect. You look exactly how you have always wanted to look. And any time you look in this beautiful mirror you can see only your ideal size and weight. And when you look at that reflection of yourself, you feeling so happy from the inside. And you are looking at yourself properly. You are noticing your marvellous posture, your beautiful facial expressions, and you can't help but notice that feeling of pride and confidence that you have felt before. And now that feeling is etched forever. You look in the mirror and you like what you see and deep inside you realise that you have worked so much hard to get here. But for now on, you will find it easy and effortless, because this is so engrained in the depth of your mind that is healthy and ideal for you. And if your mind wanders, let it be, and if you feel sleepy, don't force yourself to stay awake because your subconscious mind is listening.

[5 seconds]

You have a holistic approach towards health and you take care of yourself in all the aspects of life not just the eating healthy. Your mind is full of positive and good thoughts. You say nice and kind words to yourself. You know that you deserve the best care for yourself. And you also know that you are the only person who can take the best care of yourself. And all this magical change is happening right now. Your new personality will grow with each day. And you will notice that the change is gradual and smooth. You will enjoy the journey as well as the destination. And you will notice how far you have come. And if your mind wanders, let it be, and if you feel sleepy, don't force yourself to stay awake because your subconscious mind is listening. You will appreciate the efforts, the struggle and the changes they bring. Positive changes are visible in your health, wellbeing, physique and fitness. And from this moment on, you will be doing everything possible to make sure that you are always healthy, joyful, and happy.

[5 seconds]

You respect your miraculous body. You love the way your body is responding positively to your efforts. There are so many positive ideas floating in your mind now. You can feel the hope. You know results are around the corner. You know you will eat properly, mindfully, and will respect your food.

[5 seconds]

You eat only when you are not doing anything else. And you eat while sitting down. From now on, you will enjoy your food more than ever. Every bite, every morsel that goes in your mouth, you are going to chew it properly. You will be mindful while eating. You will take in the nourishment the food has to offer. You will enjoy the taste of what you eat. You enjoy the textures, the flavours and the smells. Your taste buds enjoy each and every bite. You think only about the food that is in your mouth. You put all your attention on to the food without any distraction on the food that is in your mouth.

[5 seconds]

You will never again feel any feelings of guilt for what you eat because you know you are now completely in control. You listen to the signals of your stomach and you stop eating when you are full. It doesn't really matter if there is food in your plate or not. You will not put the extra food in your mouth. That food which could have added fat to your body, you will let it remain on the plate. You can eat it again when you will be hungry later. But now, you just refuse to consume it. You don't feel the need or the urge to eat it. When you realise that you have eaten enough, you simply stop. And you feel extremely happy and grateful for the wonderful meal that you just enjoyed.

[5 seconds]

From now on, you will think about food only when your body needs nourishment. And if there is any time in the day when you think about eating food when you are not hungry, you have a very simple way of dealing with it. It is the same exercise that you practiced just now. You just think of that mirror you see your perfect self-looking back at you and you know that you are becoming more and more like your ideal self and merging with that image. And then you need not worry about the food. Your subconscious mind can identify if the hunger is physical or emotional. From now on, you will only eat when you are physically hungry.

[5 seconds]

From now on, whenever you feel bored and sad, you will not open the fridge or look in the kitchen to satisfy your emotional hunger. These feelings of boredom and sadness will simply fade away when you realise that they have nothing to do with your physical hunger. You are completely in control. You are happy with the way you manage everything, the way you think about food. You are so proud of your new shape and size. You are proud that your efforts have shown results. From now on, every day you will look into the mirror and you will be merging with your ideal self more and more. You appreciate the way you look. You are in love with the person you are. With each passing day, you are merging more and more with the image in the mirror – the image of an ideal you. And you feel so confident about yourself, about your body now.

The healthier, fitter you is a reality. With each passing day, you are becoming more and more one with this reality. You are turning into the ideal, the fit, the slim, the perfect version of you.

Rapid Weight Loss Gastric Band Hypnosis: Self-Hypnosis, Guided Meditations& Affirmations For Extreme Fat Burning, Food Addiction, Healthy Habits, Confidence, Anxiety& Overthinking

By Meditation Made Effortless

Copyright © 2021

All rights reserved.

No material in this book is to be utilized, reproduced in any electronic form, including recording, photocopying without permission from the author.

Table of Contents

Introduction 199

Induction 200

Relaxation Visualisation 202

Virtual Gastric Band Script 206

Portion Control.. 211

Discover the Power of Water.. 215

Raise Your Self Esteem 217

Self-Image and Attractiveness... 219

Appreciating Weight Loss 226

Exercise More... 228

Body Returning to Good Health 233

More Weight Loss 234

Stop Overanalyzing.. 237

Stop Eating Carbs 239

Manage Your Anxiety Better 241

Become More Confident 243

Script for Ego Strengthening and Success 244

Boost Happiness 246

Affirmations... 248

To the Narrator

Introduction – 12 min long

Induction – 15 min long

Relaxation Visualisation – 25 min long

Virtual Gastric Band – 25 min long

Portion Control – 25 min long

Discover the Power of Water – 25 min long

Raise Your Self Esteem -12 min long

Self-Image and Attractiveness – 15 min long

Appreciating Weight Loss – 15 min long

Exercise More – 25 min long

Body Returning to Good Health – 25 min long

More Weight Loss - 20 min long

Stop Overanalysing – 15 min long

Stop Eating Carbohydrates – 10 min long

Manage Your Anxiety Better – 15 Min long

Become More Confident – 10 min long

Script for Ego Strengthening and Success – 15 min long

Boost Happiness – 15 min long

Affirmations – 60 min long

"…" means take a breath while speaking before you continue.

PAUSE (for a few breaths)

LONGER PAUSE (give time to allow the listener time to imagine what you've suggested)

Introduction

Thank you for listening to   Rapid Weight Loss Gastric Band Hypnosis: Self-Hypnosis, Guided Meditations& Affirmations For Extreme Fat Burning, Food Addiction, Healthy Habits, Confidence, Anxiety& Overthinking.

The very fact that you have chosen to listen to this audio means that you are taking a big step on your self-love journey. And now that you have tuned in to this audio, it shows how aware of your weight related issues you are and how committed you are to losing weight and feeling happy, vibrant, and full of energy. And hypnosis can help you get an effortless head-start through this audio.

Pause

At any time when our emotions tend to overwhelm us, the first instinct we have is to feel better, to feel lighter, and to feel happier. So, in such circumstances we look for something that could comfort us and give us the opportunity to let go of the stress and anxiety that comes with overwhelming emotions. And in those moments, we turn to food to feel better.

By listening to this audio clip on a regular basis, you will be able to not just improve your awareness of the emotions you feel but you will also be able to address emotional eating. Additionally, this audio will also help you rewire your mind with the help of affirmations.

Pause

Getting a good night's sleep comes with a plethora of benefits. When you have slept well and slept enough during the night, you are able to feel energetic and productive the following morning. With such a great start to your day, you start to feel happier and more motivated to get things done, especially the things that are really important like achieving your daily diet and exercise goals to help you lose undesirable weight faster.

Congratulations to you on beginning your journey to overcome sleep and weight related issues that have been holding you back from living your best life. Each time you tune into this audio, you become more focused and feel more motivated to improve the quality of your life by improving the quality of your sleep.

Take a moment here to find yourself a comfortable spot to sit or lay down in. Make sure it's a place free from distractions. Do remember to not listen to this audio when you are moving or engaged in any activity that requires your undivided attention. And now, just make yourself comfortable.

Pause

I would also like to encourage you to use headphones so you can focus more easily on the sound of my voice as we progress.

Induction

You are now comfortable and listening to the sound of my voice... with each passing moment, you become more and more attentive to the words I say... every sound other than the sound of my voice is just the sound of everyday life that can neither disturb nor distract you but make you more attentive to the sound of my voice... and as you continue to listen to the sound of my voice you begin to feel more and more relaxed.

Pause

And now, take a deep breath in slowly letting it fill your lungs... hold your breath to a count of five... and then gently exhale through the mouth.

Pause

Let us begin...

Take another deep breath in.

Pause

Hold your breath to a count of five... one... two... three... four... five...

And now, slowly exhale... that's right.

Pause

Let's repeat this once again by taking a deep breath in...

Now hold... one...two... three... four... five.

Release and exhale gently.

Pause

One more time, take a deep breath in...

Hold... one... two... three... four... five...

Let go... exhale slowly.

Pause

You can now return to your regular pace of breath.

Pause

And now as you get comfortable with the rhythm of your breath, gently close your eyes... and as you close your eyes, slowly begin to draw your attention to the middle of your eyebrows... try to focus on this spot between your eyebrows through your mind's eye... that's right.

Pause

There is a part of you that is very creative and imaginative... a part that is so powerful that it can help you imagine anything and everything simply with the aid of your mind's eye... and I know that you can channel this creativity and imagination with ease...

Pause

I am aware that, just like the rest of us, you too have at times have found yourself drifting away in a daydream... and it is all because of the power of the part of you that's so creative, isn't it?

With the help of this part of you, you can effortlessly visualise or imagine just about anything... you can draw or paint any picture in your mind by channeling this powerful imagination in you... and in a few moments, I am going to begin talking to this powerfully creative and imaginative part of you today.

Pause

Relaxation Visualisation

And now that you have made yourself comfortable, I would like you to slowly bring your eyelids together and close your eyes. The moment you close your eyes you feel a heavy relaxation overcoming your entire body.

Pause

I want you to now draw your attention to the rhythm of your breath, concentrating on the air that you breathe in and how every inhale makes your chest expand, and how each time you exhale, the air moving out of your lungs makes your chest collapse. The more you pay attention to this rhythm, the more relaxed you feel, and the more relaxed you feel, the clearer your mind becomes, letting go of everything else and just being here in this moment.

Pause

And now, I would like you to take three deep breaths, starting with a slow inhale through your nose, focusing on the air as you breathe it in… is it warm or cool… what's the texture like… feel your lungs fill up to the brim, feel the urgency to exhale before finally letting out the air gently through your mouth. That's right.

Pause

Take one more deep breath in, same as before, and feel the air bringing in relaxation to every nook and corner of your body… feel how exhaling takes away every bit of tension from your muscles, leaving you twice more relaxed than before.

Pause

Now take one more deep breath in… noticing the relaxation in your body multiplying tenfold with each passing moment, and how the exhale brings stillness and clarity into your mind… you're so deeply relaxed now. That's right… and you're in a quiet place with the sound of my voice guiding you… making you feel even more relaxed.

Pause

It is now time to sink even deeper into this peaceful and relaxing state of mind… visualise yourself standing right outside the door of an amazing home in the mountains… this is your home amid the stunning mountains that rise up around this place… look around and notice all the tall mountainous trees... fir trees, pine trees, spruce trees... all around your home as you find yourself standing in your driveway.

Pause

Notice how the snow sits snug onto these trees... it has snowed a lot lately... It feels like a winter wonderland. You are nicely bundled up in a thick winter jacket and a warm muffler keeping you nice and warm... you have just finished shoveling snow so you look around your driveway to ensure you didn't miss any spot.

You turn to look at your house and are in awe of its beauty... it's a nice green and brown colour, blending almost entirely into the backdrop of the mountains and trees, except where the snow makes it stand out.

You now begin walking towards your front door... halfway to the door, you spot a fluffy brown rabbit hopping away in a hurry into the bushes nearby... it puts a smile on your face, relaxing you further as you reach your front porch and wipe off the excess snow off your boots.

Pause

You make your way to a chair on the porch where you sit down to take off your boots... as you take the boots off one by one and stretch your toes, they feel a little cold and you look forward to getting them warmed up.

Pause

You get up to place your boots in the shoe rack before making your way into your house which feels nice and cosy... the carpet beneath your feet is soft and incredibly warming as you walk across the room to the stone fireplace to start a fire and warm up the house... your house has large glass windows to let the natural light in...

Pause

You have done this so many times before that it seems like your hands move without you even noticing how you got the fire started... so you step back from it and notice how a spark turns into a small fire, burning up the twigs, and slowly making its way towards the bigger logs... you can notice the blue colour at the bottom of the flames... the red and orange and bright yellow colours of the flames above... as the fire grows, you can hear it crackling... it is finally starting to get warmer in your home... you can smell the burning wood... the soft scent of smoke fills up the air around you... you're feeling warmer and more relaxed... you make your way to sit on a cosy and comfortable couch beside one of the windows near the fireplace...

Pause

There's a jute basket lying beside you with a soft blanket in it... you wrap yourself in the blanket and feel nice and snug... feeling deeply relaxed and calm in the body and the mind... as you look through the windows, you can notice the majesty of the snow-clad mountains and trees... as you look further into the mountains you can notice some smoke curling up from behind some trees on a neighbouring mountain... someone else too is keeping warm by the fireplace just like you...

Pause

You begin to notice a sound in some distance... it is a familiar sound... it is the sound of a small airplane flying past the mountains, its sound echoing in the air before you can see it... the airplane is yellow in colour... you have seen plenty such airplanes in these mountains... you guess it can seat four people including the pilot... it flies away into the distance and the revving sounds of its engine too begin to fade away with it...

As you sit cosily wrapped up in a blanket beside the window, you find yourself relaxing twice as much with each sight, sound, and smell that surrounds you... you sink in further into the couch... resting your neck and your head on a soft pillow behind you... you feel such a heavy sense of relaxation filling you up... soak in all this serenity as you lie here on this cosy couch... stretching your legs just a little to feel them relax more deeply... you are nice and warm... you continue to let this relaxation sink in deeper with each passing moment.

Lying here on this couch, snug and warm beside the fireplace and the window, you are feeling so deeply relaxed. And in a few moments you will become even more relaxed.

You turn your gaze to look outside the window... you can see the snow clad trees and mountains all around... as you shift your gaze from this gorgeous scenery towards the sky above, you notice the clouds... it is about to start snowing... and looking close enough you're able to spot the first snowflakes making their way down... they are so light and beautiful... you are awed by the beauty of nature that makes these little snowflakes with such detail... the symmetry and uniqueness of each one from the other... it makes you feel more relaxed.

And now you have fixed your gaze on one particular snowflake that is a little high up in the sky and is beginning to make its way down to the ground... you feel twice as relaxed just watching it... and now as I count you down from 10 down to zero, with each count this feeling of relaxation will become heavier and heavier, sinking deeper and deeper into you, making you feel as light as this snowflake floating in the air.

Ten... you can see the snowflake moving down and down.

Nine... you are feeling twice more relaxed now.

Eight... the snow is falling down and down.

Seven... you can feel the relaxation sinking deeper and deeper.

Six... the snowflake is so close to the ground, going down and down... further and further.

Five... you can sense a heavy relaxation moving deeper and deeper into your mind and your body.

Four... you can see the snow floating all the way down, getting closer to falling into a fluffy white blanket, down and down.

Three... you are sinking deeper and deeper into this heavy state of relaxation... feeling lighter and safer.

Two... you will become more deeply relaxed than ever before when I say the next number.

One... you are fully relaxed. You are enjoying every bit of this peaceful state of relaxation... you feel you are ready now to bring about positive and constructive changes into your life.

Virtual Gastric Band Script

You are imaginative and it's so natural for you to imagine what I am going to ask you to imagine. I wonder if you could imagine that you are seeing

yourself standing at the door of the clinic -- a place where the gastric band procedures are performed. The door is right in front of you. You are feeling relaxed and confident. You turn the doorknob around and push the door open. You can see everything and everyone inside the clinic. You take the first step in and as soon as you enter the clinic, you feel safe and happy. This is an act of self-love, you're here to let go of all the extra weight that you have been carrying with you.

Pause

The clinic is quite well-known and reputed, so you know you'll be safe and that your health will be taken care of effectively and efficiently here. It is time for you to finally be a new you!

Pause

Now that you are in the clinic, you turn your gaze around slowly looking around you, seeing the different departments, doctors, nurses, and other people. You find the reception area and as you walk towards it, you are greeted by two very warm and friendly people, a man and a woman. They handle the inquiries of people who have come to the clinic to know more about the procedure, or to consult the doctors here, or get a gastric band placed on their stomach

Pause

There is a line of people just like you, queueing up at the reception area, and you follow suit... you go and stand behind the last person in line awaiting your turn. As you stand here waiting, you continue to look around yourself and notice the staff of the clinic moving about... you can see how hard-working and friendly they are... they are handling everything with great professionalism... you can see they are adept at their job and skilled in the delivery and fulfilment of their services.

Pause

You begin to move ahead in the queue until it's finally your turn... you reach the desk and hear the receptionist saying, "Hello Sir (or Ma'am, depending on your client's gender)! How may I assist you?" You hand over the papers you have containing the details of your appointment with the doctor today... after checking your papers, the receptionist takes you along to guide you towards the general room of the clinic at the end of a corridor... you enter the room and look around to see a bed white fresh white sheets and some clothes... as you walk towards the bed, your doctor's assistant walks in to ask you to get dressed in the clothes lying on the bed.

Pause

Once the assistant leaves, you change your clothes and lie down on the bed... it is a very comfortable bed that makes you feel cozy and relaxed... you are now waiting for the doctor to call you in to get the procedure started.

Pause

While you wait, a nurse walks into your room... she is very warm and friendly... She tells you that she is here to talk to you about the gastric band procedure in detail.

Pause

She talks to you in detail about the procedure, going over the fact that it is an absolutely non-invasive process that involves placing a silicone band around your stomach to help restrict the amount of food you consume... she takes her time to slowly explain the rest... especially how placing this band will simply affect the amount of food you eat and nothing else.

Pause

With the help of the kind nurse, you learn that placing the silicone band around your stomach will reduce its size to that of a golf ball, allowing you to eat only small portions of food... this means you will be able to shed weight faster and more efficiently...

Pause

Being a non-invasive procedure, it will be completely safe, healthy, and natural for you... you will be able to easily lose any unwanted or extra weight from your body... and you will be able to do so from the moment the band is placed around your stomach, more so when you supplement it with consistent exercise and a healthy diet... you know you can do it... you understand the procedure very well now.

Pause

Having acquainted you with the procedure, the nurse smiles as she gets up to leave the room... before leaving, she informs you that the doctor will be with you in another few minutes.

Pause

Now that the nurse has left, you take a deep breath in, filling yourself with more relaxation and then letting out a slow and deep exhale... you know the procedure completely now... you feel more empowered with the knowledge that it is absolutely safe and non-invasive... you feel motivated already to eat consciously and exercise daily to reap the benefits of this procedure.

Pause

The doctor's assistant enters the room and asks you to follow him towards the procedure room... you get up from the bed and proceed to follow him... you notice yourself slowly walking past various other rooms... in one such room on your left, you see a man (or a woman, as per the gender of your client) laying on a bed surrounded by family... you notice that s/he is very overweight... you stop to look closely and see his/her arms, legs, and belly... you can feel they are filled with lots of fat and sludge... you wonder if s/he is dying... you then notice someone walking out of that room, crying... you walk up to them to inquire what's wrong with the man/woman in the room... The man/woman's wife (or husband or any other person As per your client's family) tells you that s/he is lying on her/his deathbed because of obesity... s/he is here because s/he overate and could not control him/herself due to which s/he is dying now... the doctors have told them that s/he only has a few more hours of life left...

Pause

You may find yourself wondering about the negative consequences of being overweight... that's alright, it's okay to wonder... however, what happened to the man/woman in that room is not going to happen to you... with the help of the virtual gastric band, put right in time via a non-invasive process, you will be able to shed the extra weight and feel satiated with smaller portions of food, leading you closer to a slimmer and healthier version of yourself so soon.

Visualization

You now begin to follow the doctor's assistant once again... making your way slowly behind him as he leads you to the procedure room... you find yourself entering a big room which feels very comfortable and secure... there is a bed that the assistant gestures for you to lie down on while you wait patiently for the doctor to arrive... meanwhile, the assistant calls an anaesthetist.

Pause

As the anaesthetist enters the room alongside the surgeon, they both greet you with a warm smile that makes you feel relaxed and comfortable... before the procedure can start, the assistant hands over a consent form for you to sign... you go through the details mentioned on the form and understand fully and completely that in order to achieve permanent, natural, and safe weight-loss, you need to drink plenty of water, eat healthy food, and exercise regularly... you then sign the consent form and hand it back to the assistant, who then leaves the procedure room.

Pause

The anaesthetist begins talking to you, asking you about how important it is for you to lose weight and what the new you would look like... and slowly and gradually you begin drifting further and further, deeper and deeper, the sounds around you fading away into the distance...

Pause

And now, I wonder if you can notice what the size and shape of your stomach is... you can now notice a silicone gastric band being placed around your stomach... you can notice the size of your stomach shrinking slowly... until it acquires the size of a golf ball... that's right... your stomach is now the size of a small golf ball that could easily fit into the palm of your hand... a small sized stomach that can only accommodate small portions of healthy, nutritious food... you also notice that the band is tightened just enough to allow smaller portions of food to fill it, without depriving you of the pleasure of eating... and the band will stay this way for a long time to come.

Pause

The procedure has been a great success... the band has been securely fit around your stomach and there are no scars left behind... it was completely non-invasive... the surgeon now proceeds to remove all the equipment... you look absolutely fine and feel wonderful already.

Pause

This gastric band has successfully reduced the size of your stomach... it can even be adjusted or removed in the future if need be.

Pause

You begin drifting deeper and deeper... soaking in the blissful feelings of success and the excitement and motivation to get started on your journey towards healthy and natural weight loss...

You visualise yourself three months from now with this gastric band placed around your stomach... you get acquainted with your body that has shed a lot of weight... you notice yourself from head to toe... notice how you look... notice how you feel... and when you step outside, notice how people are so surprised and cheerful seeing you... let these feelings sink in deeper and deeper now.

Pause

As you continue to look at and notice this future self of yours... this slimmer and healthier version of yourself... I am sure you can easily recount all the important steps you took consciously and confidently to reach here in these three months... were you eating consciously, were you chewing your food effectively, were you getting more exercise regularly? Allow all of these feelings and all the answers to sink in deeper and deeper.

Direct Suggestions

From this moment on, this gastric band works for your best interests and benefit...
You are conscious about what you eat and how you eat it... you chew each mouthful properly whilst enjoying the flavours and textures...
You consume smaller portions of food that make your golf ball sized stomach feel satisfied and full easily every single day, in every single meal...
You exercise daily and feel motivated to achieve your goals...
You feel inspired and look forward to each new day with a renewed sense of purpose to achieve your desirable weight...
You deeply and completely love yourself inside-out...
All these suggestions continue to become stronger with each passing moment and each passing hour...

Pause

You are now becoming aware of your surroundings in the procedure room... regaining awareness of the sights and sounds around you... the nurse greets you with a huge smile as she proceeds to inform you about how successful the procedure was... and listening to say this, makes you feel so deeply relaxed and elated... you feel confident that you're one step closer to becoming a slimmer and healthier you... you are perfectly alright and ready to head home... so you slowly get up from this bed and make your way to the general room where your clothes are... you reach the general room and change your clothes.

Portion Control

I want you to simply lay down with your eyes closed, relax your body and lay comfortably with your legs and hands crossed. I want you to focus on your breaths. I want you to become aware of each breath that you inhale and each breath that you exhale. You are going good, with each breath out, just imagine.....breathing out all that does have any purpose....I know you are capable enough to do this...because everybody can do this....and....so....just take a deep breath in and then breath out...all the unwanted thoughts.....you are doing good. Focus on the feeling of the rise of your chest....and when you breath out...focus on how your chest falls...that is correct....let your hands, legs and arms loosen up...making them relaxed....comfortable.....and at peace. You relax and then you relax even more....as you keep on listening to my voice...each breath relaxed you even more...allowing you to escape away...into a different state of mind...magical to be precise...allowing you to be more comfortable, calm, quiet and relaxed....that is right....

(Deepener)

Now I want you to imagine a staircase anywhere....it could either be in a building or a garden or at any other place that your subconscious mind is allowing you to be...now imagine yourself going down that staircase of 10 steps....and each step that you take brings you twice as deep....calming you even more....more than ever.....so...10...9.....becoming more relaxed and at ease....8.....7....enjoying the feeling of going down....at....6...5...allow yourself to relax more than before......4......3....tell yourself....that you are going deeper and deeper and deeper...2.......more and more relaxed......and 1......0.

Now I am wondering if you could think of all the reasons that made you want to lose weight...just think about it....all of that right now...certainly....you may want yourself at your ideal weight....and goal size. And it's normal to wonder, just let all that come right into your mind.

Perhaps...wearing your favourite outfit and dressing, walking and talking confidently with your family, relatives, friends and colleagues...you have a high amount of confidence, high self-esteem....and all that falls in the right place in front of you...just think about all those right now.

My grandfather had once told me that you are born with a natural inbuilt ability to know what you can do and that if you have had enough.

And as you live your life and go through everyday events, you usually tend to ignore the signals that your body is conveying to stop eating or working out. When you ignore such signals you eat more in a huge quantity, this results in stomach expansion...adding more weight to your body...which ultimately results in a person who has low self-esteem, low confidence and is lethargic.

But now since you have finally decided to stop overeating and become the confident and strong person that you have always wanted to be. The time has now come to change your eating pattern as well.

(Metaphor)

I am wondering if you know that infants eat so less and they have a small stomach than we do. However, when they start eating more, their stomach expands and that means that they are willing to eat more....

And, if you want you can reverse this process as well, eat less to make your stomach smaller...

And, I am wondering....if you could simply go back...becoming younger and fitter....to your teenage days...becoming more and more younger.....maybe to the young age of...

10...9....and then maybe even 7....going back....to the age of 5....and then 4....to the early years...when you used to eat less....even less than what you eat now....perhaps to the age of two years...when your stomach was very small and you ate so less...
Experience all those feelings now.

(Pause)

I am wondering if you can now connect yourself to that time... subconsciously...just try to make a connection in whatever way possible...and your subconscious mind will know it all...so...try to make a connection right now...become that person with the feeling of eating less...and leaving some extra food in the bowl...the time when you were full and happy enough with small amount of food.

(Pause)

Connect yourself.

Now try to make a bridge from that time up to now...and imagine yourself talking steps...slowly...towards the present time...now imagine yourself taking slow steps...towards the present....walking on the bridge...looking down.....perhaps looking at yourself...at a distance...from far away...seeing yourself...your body...and...shape...that you do not like it now...but from far away....from the bridge...and as you keep on moving on the bridge....you will realise that...you now have a small stomach...a stomach of a baby...that can only eat in small quantities.....perhaps...a stomach of the size of a ball....so small that you can even hold it in your palms...a small stomach...that can get full by eating in small amounts...making you feel content after few mouthfuls.

(Pause for about 30 seconds)

And as you come back to the present times...to the present second...feeling the new shrunken stomach in your body....feel it...experience it....you already know that you can just hold the right amount of food in there...you must feel full at the right time to be able to shed off those extra mass and to get back to the right shape and size.

Now I am wondering if you could imagine yourself at a table with food right in front of you on a plate...and as you see that...you ask....can I eat all this?

You start eating and as you eat, you chew the food slowly, perhaps about 15-20 times...enjoying every bite with flavours.

Your stomach is as small as the size of a ball...and it has shrunken...making your stomach look flat and toned...with each passing day your tummy is becoming flattered, fitter and smaller...as you are eating less and feeling more satisfied.

With each passing second, you are realising that you have more energy, more enthusiasm, high confidence and high self-esteem.

(Future Goal Setting)

I am wondering if you could imagine yourself 6 months from now....when you have shed those extra fats...feeling fitter, healthier and stronger.

You are having a nice glow on your face, you can get into your desired clothes' size, you can even inspire others...as you are having a perfect body that everyone desires......

And suddenly one day you get a call for dinner gets together from someone who has not seen you from the past 6 months...so you decide to get into your favourite dress, drive down, walking towards their house.

You ring the bell and when they open the door they...they look shocked about how beautiful and amazing you look. They even say – O M G...is this you? How amazing you look. You look so much better, you look fit and so slim. And you say with full confidence- THANK YOU.

You get into their house and move towards the table where dinner is to be served

And you see that the plate has only that amount of food which you can very easily consume. Which can be very easily taken by your small stomach. You start chewing the food properly, slowly and slowly, about 15-20 times, enjoying the flavours...savouring each mouth full.

And this is the time when you realise that your appetite has drastically reduced, large portions of the meal do not interest you- you don't need it- you don't want it.

This is making you feel good- you are feeling that you are in control of your mind, body and health.

These suggestions are engraved in your subconscious mind and are making you grow stronger day by day.

They grow stronger every second, of every minute, of every hour, of every day.
In a moment I am going to count numbers from one to five and by the count of five, you will be fully alert and refreshed- ready for the suggestion to work for you.

Discover the Power of Water

You continue to relax deeper and deeper... feeling more and more relaxed.

With your mind's eye, I would like you to visualise your body as a glass cylinder... you can now see that there is some crystal clear water with magical and healing properties beginning to pour into this cylinder... the water starts to pour in through the very top of your head... and this magical healing water makes its way right down to your feet...

Pause

Filling you up starting from the bottom of your feet and toes... making you feel warm and soothed... slowly filling up your body moving up into your shins and calves... relaxing and healing and soothing your knees, thighs and hips... providing you nourishment, care, and hydration as it begins to fill up your waist, abdomen, stomach and chest... you can feel its healing energy rushing through every part of you as it fills up your chest and begins to move into your shoulders, your arms, your wrists, and your fingers... calming you... relaxing you... removing all toxins and unhelpful substances from your body as it begins to fill up your neck, your chin, your cheeks, your eyes, your ears, your forehead... all the way up to the top of your head... and now, every cell, muscle, fibre and bone in your body is filled with this crystal clear healing water... this magical water has cleansing properties... so, relax even further... and notice how this water begins to gently become warmer... as the water becomes warmer, it charges up each and every cell of your body, activating the cells , cleansing them, and healing them.

Pause

As the magic of the water begins to unfold throughout your body, imagine water as the best antioxidant... water is the best antioxidant as it cleanses your body right down to the cellular level

Pause

You can feel your body aligning in perfect harmony with itself... as your body enters this perfect harmony with itself, it also aligns in perfect harmony with its environment and everything that surrounds it... simply by reaping the benefits from the power of water.

Pause

The water continues to warm a little more... and as the water gets warmer, you feel more and more relaxed and at ease... you can easily feel the energy reverberate through every cell in your body... as each cell has now been cleansed and healed... the cells of your body have been rid of toxins and more room has been made for nutrition to flow into them... all the toxic substances that were doing your body harm have been done away with... and this process is continuing even now... the magical healing water begins to work even harder to cleanse your body and bring natural healing to every part of your body... you can feel this process happening naturally and continuing even long after the conclusion of this hypnotherapy session... you can feel the water restoring your body, each and every cell in it to its natural glory... you can feel the water repairing any damage, removing all toxicity, and restoring health.

Pause

I would now like you to visualise that at the bottom of each feet, there is some liquid beginning to drain away from your body... just like the process of changing the oil in a car... the oil is poured in, it moves through the engine, cleansing it, lubricating it, draining out and carrying all impurities with it... and then it needs to be changed.

Pause

In a similar fashion, the water entering your body has cleansed it, healed it, restored its health, and is now draining out of it carrying with it all the toxins and impurities with it... which is why the liquid draining from the bottom of your feet looks dirty...

Pause

Your body has now been cleaned... and each time you repeat this process, your body becomes cleaner and healthier...

Pause

And now that your body has been cleaned, it begins to fill up with lots of natural energy... this energy can be of any colour you choose it to be... it slowly fills up each and every part of your body helping you soak in the magic of water to the fullest.

Pause

You can now fully gauge the power of water... you now ensure that each time you find yourself feeling thirsty, you drink water... because you know now that it's the best form of liquid for your body and wellbeing... you not just drink water, but enjoy it too... you know it's vital for your health as it helps repair and rejuvenate your body... it helps rid your body of substances that are toxic and unhelpful for you... you are now developing habits that are healthy and helpful for you...

Pause

you are eating food that is healthy and nutritious for you... you are drinking more water and staying hydrated... you are avoiding unhealthy food and drinks... you are choosing to exercise every day... you are keeping your mind positive and thoughts constructive... you are finding yourself taking more interest in what you have faith in and thereby catering to your spiritual health as well... you are noticing how your mind, body and soul are aligning in perfect harmony... you are becoming more and more healthy with each passing day.

Your body has now been suggested to be in perfect health... you are now relaxing more and more.

216

Raise Your Self Esteem

Now, I want you to slowly drift into a deep relaxation, and in this relaxed state of mind, I want you to realise just how powerful you are, and I want you to realise that you are an amazing, and a wonderful person.

Imagine yourself standing in front of a mirror looking at yourself, and take a close look.

Pause

Notice all the attractive qualities you possess.

And with continuous practise, you will slowly begin to realise how much easier it is for you to notice more and more such beautiful qualities about yourself.

You will realise how smart, attractive, and intelligent you are.

Pause

Everyone around you easily notices these qualities as well.

They can easily see that you are attractive, smart, and intelligent.

Your beauty and positivity shines through.

Pause

Now I would like you to think of three qualities about yourself that make you unique.

It could be how kind you are, or it could be your strength to persevere, or even just how positive you are.

So, go ahead and notice these three wonderful and unique things about yourself.

And with the help of this recording, you will find it easier and easier to notice these qualities.

Pause

Now, take a deep breath, and as you inhale, imagine all the positivity and confidence entering your body, and as you exhale, let all the negative thoughts leave you.

Let your breath flow easily and effortlessly.

Pause

With each passing day, your self-esteem is improving, and you are beginning to realise your full potential.

You are very powerful, attractive and intelligent.

You have a limitless bag of wonderful qualities.

Pause

And as you begin to notice more and more of these wonderful qualities, you realize how great you feel about yourself.

You feel a powerful sense of self-love, and you use all of this positive energy in the most productive way possible.

Pause

You are kind to others as you are kind to yourself.

You respect yourself, and therefore you are careful to avoid negative situations. You make better decisions, and you only put yourself in situations which honor you.

This helps you in building your confidence, will-power and self-esteem immensely.

It makes you feel wonderful.

Pause

You eat right, exercise regularly, you have fun, and you are enjoying life.

You do all of this because you respect yourself, and you therefore look after the well-being of your mind and body.

Pause

These positive and wonderful activities help you build a powerful sense of self-esteem.

Self-Image and Attractiveness

Now, allow yourself to enter a deep relaxed state where you feel a complete sense of calmness.

And, in this relaxed state, keep your mind open to all the positive suggestions I am about to share with you.

These positive suggestions are going to benefit you in abundance, and these benefits will be permanent.

Pause

But before we go deeper into the suggestions, I want you to first realise that you are a kind person, and you have many loveable qualities which is why everyone around finds you to be a warm, charming personality.

You are full of life, fun-to-be-around, and a happy-go-lucky kind of person.

Unfortunately, due to certain recent events, this positive side of you received a severe set-back.

And, therefore you were not able to see clearly.

Pause

The blue skies were replaced with dark and gloomy clouds which dampened your spirits, and forced you down a road of self-destruction - making it hard for you to see all the beautiful qualities you have to offer.

But the fact is that you are an intelligent, bright individual who is well aware that attractiveness and self -love is a state of mind, and this cannot be experienced by buying expensive hair products or make-up.

These products can only help you change your appearance which at best is a momentary satisfaction.

Pause

It is therefore more fruitful to channelize your energies in feeling better on the inside first, and then once you are in a better frame of mind, you will see how this positivity automatically helps you look better.

You carry a certain vibrancy and enthusiasm with you.

Now, I want you to take a moment and think about all the people you consider to be attractive.

It could be anyone including friends, family, acquaintances or even celebrities.

Now, notice their posture, smile, and clear skin, and understand that these qualities are a result of their confidence and overall positivity.

Pause

In simple words, because they feel good, they look good, and so the cycle continues.

So, it really just boils to believing in yourself, cause if you believe in yourself, you will feel good inside, you will be upbeat and vibrant, and these positive energies will in turn change your appearance and make you look good.

Pause

In fact, if you go deeper and observe closely, you will see how a simple smile on a person's face can change your perception of their appearance.

Another fascinating trait is to do with belief.

As you begin to believe more in your abilities, the more you continue to grow in confidence which then helps you push beyond the boundaries that you once perceived.

Pause

So now, as you believe more in your attractiveness and beautiful qualities, you will radiate with confidence, and the people around you will notice this and compliment you, and you will have faith in their compliments because of your confidence.

As you can now see, these patterns and cycles are almost self-fulfilling in several different ways, and as you keep going, it gets better and better.

Now, I want you to use your imagination and let your mind be immersed into a deep state of hypnosis.

I can see that you have achieved a deep state of relaxation, and I can see you enjoying this state of mind.

Pause

Now, I want you to know that as you begin to use your imagination in this state of mind, you will be exercising the same parts of your brain just as it would in real circumstances.

It is therefore vital that you let yourself really feel good.

So feel the best you can, become a master of your own happiness so that when you wake from this hypnosis, these feelings become a natural state of mind to you.

Now let your imagination float a little further, and imagine yourself in the presence of a person you consider to be attractive or someone you look up to.

Make a note of their physical presence, their posture and other positive characteristics that stand out.

Now imagine yourself stepping into this person's body, and let yourself feel as attractive as you imagine them to be.

Notice how this sensation immediately lifts your spirits.

Pause

Take a few steps around and enjoy the posture, the stride, eyes bright and wide, head held high.

Now, I want you to pay close attention to your breath, and observe where in your body you sense these good sensations, and notice how these sensations move within your body.

Stay with me as we go a further into this sensation, and I want you think of a colour that would symbolize this feeling of confidence and attractiveness.

Now, imagine yourself standing tall and being bathed in this special colour.

Imagine yourself smiling, feeling attractive and let yourself really feel good.

Pause

Now, gently squeeze your thumb against your finger, and know that you are now aware of all the secrets to looking and feeling good.

Repeat this several times.

Now that you have familiarized yourself with all these wonderful sensations, you will find it easy to revisit these feelings as and when you feel the need to simply by squeezing your thumb against your finger.

Now gently bring your attention back to your breath, and slowly drift out of their body, and thank the person for allowing you to feel all of those wonderful sensations.

In a few moments, I am going to reach over and lift your hand, and then I am going to give you some more suggestions and as I begin to do so, you will notice how your hands naturally start to drift down with you making any effort.

Pause

And when your hand touches your lap, it will serve as an indication of the agreement that the necessary changes have occurred in your subconscious, and with this you will notice a dramatic change in your feelings and behaviour.

You will feel an immense improvement in your overall self image, confidence, and happiness.

Now, continue to relax and let yourself sink deeper, and as you go deeper I want you to realize that no matter what you do, you will do so in a relaxed manner, and this will help you enjoy whatever it is you are doing.

You will feel comfortable, confident and in complete control in any situation.

This will build your self-esteem, and you will continue to grow in confidence and self acceptance.

Now the suggestions I am about to make will slowly drift down into your subconsciousness, and as these suggestions sink in, you will notice how you feel better about yourself.

You will find it easy to navigate difficult situations, persons or places.

And in this state of mind nothing can annoy you or disturb you.

You will be able to adjust to any situation and you will be able to achieve this with ease.

Now I want you to picture yourself in this state of mind.

Imagine how you want to be.

You will be strong, and you will be able to stand up for yourself when needed.

You will be able to state your opinion or suggestions without any embarrassment or anxiety.

Pause

And as this happens, you will grow in confidence.

You will feel a sense of vibrancy all around you.

Perfect and Radiant Health

Take a long, deep breath and let yourself sink deeper into a relaxed state of mind.

Now imagine a tall, clear glass jar with an open top.

Pay close attention to its shape and size.

Now I want you to picture yourself as the glass jar standing upright.

And imagine the top of your head to be the open mouth of the glass jar, and imagine a green liquid being poured in.

This liquid is going to cleanse your body and soothe your soul.

Observe how the liquid poured in from the top of your head runs all the way down to the bottom of your feet, and now feel the liquid slowly filling up your body from the bottom to the top.

Notice the warm, soothing sensation in the soles of your feet.

Pause

And as the liquid works its way upward to your knees, you feel a warm, cleaning and soothing sensation taking over.

You feel relaxed and at ease.

The liquid is now slowly upward toward your thighs, soothing and relaxing all of the muscles in your thighs.

Now the liquid is moving up to your lower abdomen, and as it gently fills up your waist area, you can feel your body being cleansed.

All your organs and muscles feel rejuvenated.

You can feel your chest and shoulders relax, and as the liquid oozes down your shoulders, through your biceps toward your elbow, and then down to your wrists and finger tips, your hands start to feel relaxed.

The liquid has now filled your entire body all the way up to your neck, cleansing and healing your body.

As it slowly makes its way to your cheeks, your mouth, your nose and ears, you feel a sense of relaxation and calmness take over you.

Your body is now filled from top to bottom with this relaxing, green liquid.

And the reason we chose the colour green for the liquid is because green is the colour of healing.

For example, plants are green in colour and they are full of energy.

Now, let yourself relax a little deeper, and observe how the green liquid begins to turn slightly warm as it activates every cell in your body, and as it turns warm it is also cleaning and healing your mind, body and soul.

Think of this green liquid as the perfect antioxidant, and observe how it helps your mind and body come into complete harmony with its surroundings.

Now, I want you to let yourself slowly drift deeper into a relaxed state of mind, and observe how the green liquid begins to get a little more warm with each passing second, and notice how each and every cell in your body begins to feel cleansed, healed and rejuvenated.

As you continue to work with this recording, you can choose a particular muscle, organ or any other part of your body.

You can even use this recording for just general health and wellness.

For now, let us go ahead and select a particular part of your body and work on it.

Once you have chosen a particular part of your body, observe how the warmth of the green liquid cleanses and heals that part of your body.

Let that part of your body relax deeply.

Now take a deep breath, and I want you to imagine this green liquid slowly oozing out of your toes.

Imagine this process to be similar to that of an oil change in a vehicle.

The oil goes into the engine, lubricates and cleans the engine.

Now, as the green liquid oozes out of your toes, notice that it is a little dirty as it carries all the toxin out of your body.

Each time you repeal this process, your body becomes cleaner and healthier.

Relax deeply, and notice how the green liquid has almost entirely oozed out of your body, taking all the toxins along with it, and as this takes place, observe how your body fills itself with natural energy.

You can imagine this energy to be of any colour you want.

As your body fills up with this natural energy, feel it revitalize every cell in your mind and body.

This energy will help you develop healthier eating habits. It will help you avoid unhealthy food, and help you exercise on a regular basis.

It will help you stay mentally positive and focussed.

You will be more productive, and you will take care of your spiritual health.

You will find the perfect balance, and your mind, body and soul will be in perfect harmony.

So relax and realize that everything is going to be just fine because you are becoming more and more healthy with each passing day.

Your body is now naturally in a healthy state, perfect and radiant.

Now let yourself relax deeply.

Appreciating Weight Loss

As we progress through this session, I want you to take the time and look back, and reflect on how far you have come.

Think back to the time when you first arrive here, and realize all the monumental improvements you have made, and take pride in these immense positive changes you have made.

Think back and take note of all the difficulties and setbacks you have overcome, and think of all the challenges you faced during this time, and how you did not let anything stop you from continuing your progress.

You took up the challenge of becoming slimmer and healthier, and you put in every ounce of energy into achieving this goal.

You kept your focus on your daily tasks which helped you make progress on a day to day basis while keeping in mind your larger goal, and that has helped you come such a long way.

And since you have worked so hard, you will treasure the results far more than anyone else.

You appreciate yourself and your progress a lot more because you have worked so hard for it.

To give you an example, imagine a young man who wins a million pounds in a lottery.

He may feel like all of his dreams have come true, however, such a dramatic change of lifestyle can be quite damaging in the long term.

This young man may have no time to adjust to his new lifestyle, and will most likely not value the win.

On the other hand, a man who worked everyday determined and focussed on making a million pounds will really understand and appreciate the value of this money.

With that awareness, you know that you too will have to work hard to achieve your goal but this will be something you enjoy doing as it will be beneficial for you overall.

Each day picture yourself in your new slimmer and healthier body, and know that with each passing day you are moving one step closer to your end goal.

And as you make progress with each passing day, take time to appreciate your efforts, and you can take great pride in talking yourself about all the hard-work and commitment you have put in.

And every time you think about eating food that is not conducive for your goals, you will remind yourself of all the hard work you are putting in.

Think about the way you want to look and feel, and as soon as you do that, you will automatically choose a healthier eating option.

Pause

And soon you will find that you enjoy healthier food not only because it is good for your body but also because it is more tasty and nutritious.

If at all you find yourself not eating right or there is a slight increase in your weight (and this might rarely happen), you will take it as a sign to work harder and not give up.

You will no longer have to use the phrase 'You can do it' because you already are doing it, and you will feel that energy within yourself and know exactly what it is like to be an achiever.

Pause

You will feel it now, and you will feel it growing with each passing day.

Exercise More

Now as you rest and relax, I want you to reflect on the problem that you came here with today, and along with these problems I want you to take note of all the excuses you created which ensured you continued to stay with the problem instead of finding the solution.

It is uncanny how people react when faced with a problem.

They find it more painful to make a change that will help resolve the problem but won't mind prolonging the pain that comes with leaving the problem unattended.

I want you to now take a step back to something you mentioned earlier about you needing to make a better effort of going to the gym and getting fit.

Pause

You want to make these changes but you just can't seem to find the will to do so.

But imagine a day 12 months from now, and picture yourself driving past the gym on your way home.

You deliberately keep your eyes steady on the road as if to say you did not notice the gym at all.

You can sense that you are clutching the steering wheel a little tightly, and your heart is beating faster, and this is because there is a voice inside of you that is fully aware that you should be going to the gym but somehow, you just cannot seem to put your words into action.

As you slow-down in the traffic, you notice that your clothes do not feel as comfortable. They have become tight, and it is not because your clothes have suddenly shrunk - it is because you have gained weight.

Pause

Eventually, as you get home you feel really tired and sluggish, and you have been feeling like this for a while now.

Maybe you need to relax and unwind, prepare your dinner and take a bath whilst it is cooking.

So you go into the kitchen to prepare your dinner but you are already a bit hungry so you search the fridge and the cupboards for something to snack on whilst you decide what to cook.

Pause

Since you went grocery shopping just the day before, you have plenty of food to choose from but you seem to be going through the food far more quickly these days - maybe it is because you are spending more time at home sitting around and watching television instead of exercising.

Anyway, you find a snack and prepare for dinner. It's just you in the house, and so you get ready for your bath whilst you leave the oven on to heat up.

Pause

As you begin to undress, you notice your body bursting out of the seams like a prisoner being released from jail.

You notice indents on your body. The lines of the seams of your clothes have left deep marks on your skin, and even though you briefly flirt with the thought that your clothes have shrunk, you know well that this is all because you have gained weight over the past few months.

Now, walk toward the mirror and take a close look at your body, and take a rough guess about the amount of weight you have gained over the past 12 months - ½ stone, or a whole stone, or maybe more?

Pause

Notice how your flesh seems to hang and sag, and how some other parts of your body are becoming lumpy and uneven.

You also seem to have gained weight on your face, and your cheeks look puffed up.

You are briefly struck with a sickening panic because the work that would have been simple to execute 12 months ago, now seems twice as hard to achieve.

It feels as if you have gone a step too far, like you have passed the point of no return.

You feel a growing resentment inside of you as you recall all the times that you drove past the gym, and all those times that you made excuses to not go ahead and workout.

It takes a lot of pain and effort to lose excess weight, and it always feels easier to just cover it up but you now realise that in the long run it is more painful to look at yourself in the mirror with all this excess weight, and a growing sense of hopelessness.

You abandon your bath as you cannot bear to stand and look at yourself in the flesh anymore, and you desperately search through your wardrobe for something comfortable to wear.

You wander around the house tidying up and preparing your dinner but you feel an overwhelming urge to just lay down and idle away your time.

You are well aware of the work that lies ahead but lethargy seems to be getting the better of you.

You also are well aware that this lethargy is because you have put on all this excess weight.

Now, let's take a step further and picture yourself another 12 months into the future.

It's been a tough week at work, and you are out shopping by yourself. You could have gone shopping with your friends, but they are out looking for swimwear, and you avoid them cause you can no longer wear swimsuits. You have put on far too much weight, and you feel extremely conscious about your body.

You need to shop because none of your clothes fit you anymore. You go into one of your favourite stores, and you pick up a few pieces that really excite you.

You take them to the trial to try them on but it ends up being a disastrous affair.

Firstly, you struggle tremendously to get your clothes off - it is all too tight.

Then as you finally manage to wriggle out, you find it equally hard to slip something on.

You then realize that you have grown tremendously in size. The size you estimated yourself to be was a way off the mark.

You check the labels to ensure you picked the right pieces, and to your dismay, you see that you did pick the right size.

You are finding it extremely difficult to wriggle into it but somehow you just do not want to accept it, and so you continue to struggle and wriggle your way into it.

Suddenly you realize that you have pushed it too far, and now you can't seem to get it off you - and you are now stuck with these clothes halfway through.

You start feeling really terrible, and you can feel a sudden sense of panic take over you.

Suddenly, you start feeling hot, and you notice yourself sweating profusely.

You can feel your heart pounding in your chest.

One of the sales staff senses something wrong, and is heading toward the changing room to check if you are alright.

You realize that you are deep into a panic attack, and you feel extremely embarrassed.

You realize you are going to need help to gather yourself, and so when the sales staff knocks on your door, you hesitantly let the assistant enter, and as you stand there red-faced, you explain that you are stuck and you are not able to get the clothes off of you.

You keep babbling and apologizing profusely.

The sales assistant looks equally embarrassed and hesitantly helps to free you.

Unsure what to do next, the sales assistant asks you if you would like to try on a larger size, but that makes you feel awful and low, and so with tears rolling down your eyes, you decline the offer, and you get dressed quickly and leave.

You feel sad and down, but not just because you have gained all this weight, but because you feel like all your friends and loved ones are slowly slipping away from you - you feel unloved.

The days when you once felt good about yourself is now only a distant memory.

These days you only feel disappointment and resentment, and you feel like you spend all your time wallowing in negative thoughts.

Now, take a deep breath, and slowly step away from that image, and come back to the present moment.

And I now want you to pay close attention to my voice. Let your senses follow my voice just as my voice will follow you wherever you go.

Through this journey, you have seen the difference between success and failure, and you now know exactly what it takes to be successful.

You have experienced first hand how successful people do not believe in making excuses.

Think back to a time when you felt extremely committed to something, and recall how you were indifferent to what others had to say to deter you.

No matter what obstacle came your way, it couldn't stop you from doing what you wanted to only because you were that committed to the cause.

And when you are committed to something, you really apply your mind, body and soul in achieving whatever it is you have set your eyes on.

And in this state of mind, no level of difficulty can deter you.

No matter how hard it gets, you still carry a feeling of certainty of doing what it takes to overcome the situation.

Can you recall a time like that in your life?

Can you recall those feelings?

So, you now know that you have the ability to do whatever it takes to achieve your goal, and all you have to do is to set your goal, and then commit yourself to achieving this goal.

Put your words into action, and stay focussed on taking small steps and doing the right things on a day to day basis.

The time has now come for you to take all this awareness and put it into action, and stay committed to your goal.

Body Returning to Good Health

What do you exactly see when you look into the mirror? Do you think it is you, the real you? Or is it just another created thought that prompts your subconscious mind to send a pre-programmed understanding of you, an addition of previous familiarities and conditioning. Whatever might be the answer to the question and you may have to think deeply about that, I would like to tell you that how you feel about yourself is going to change forever and for the better, to improve the quality of your life, to make you feel revived, like a gentle wind, throwing away the cobwebs that have masked your qualities and charm.

Pause

So that the confidence that you have in yourself can thrive, stronger and deeper, every second, of every minute, of every hour, of every day. Let's now change our focus on your body entirely. Your body is a very beautiful miracle of nature. How many plants and trees you know can impact their health solely by thinking positively? And how many animals you know that with the power of mind self-heal?

Pause

You can affect every single part of your body, just by thinking about it, you can make it either better or worse. This is what is called getting what you focus on. Have you ever thought of getting a new car and suddenly you see that car driven around everywhere! It's the same thing. If someone is not feeling well, it's not enough to think that 'I don't want to worry about my ailments' or 'I don't want this illness anymore' because when you think this way your mind will find the positive of those statements which will eventually result in 'I want this illness' and ' I want to worry'. From now onwards, I want you to start reviewing and censoring all the thoughts in your head and all the words from your mouth and just focus on all the good things.

I want you to say every day," My body is returning to its natural shape" and "My body looks after me very well". I do not have to worry about that. There are a lot of activities taking place inside your body without you even realizing those. Blinking, talking and walking are all-natural and automatic and I suspect that if you think about these too much, these natural and familiar functions may begin to seem quite different and unfamiliar. And if you focus more on that oddness, the more concerned you are going to become until paranoia evolves which will certainly lead to stress reactions in these parts of the body. It's a fact that your body does the best when you relax, and the more you relax the better your body functions.

I want you to make your body feel relaxed and focus on feeling well by next week. You are going to feel different about how you feel.

More Weight Loss

You are going to obtain a positive approach to get this slim, healthy and attractive body of your dreams. My suggestions are going to change the thinking about your body forever.

These small tips and ideas are going to make deep changes and thorough effect upon the deepest part of your subconscious mind, it is going to become a the permanent part of every cell of your mind and body and will remain there throughout.

These suggestions are going to be helpful and you are going to be stunned and surprised to see the effectiveness of these small sentences, they are going to be a part of your everyday life, giving you a lot of brand new patterns, thoughts, a new method of action to make you a successful and significant person.

You are going to make use of brand new methods that you have never used before. You have already begun your journey of achieving a beautiful, attractive and healthy body that you have dreamt of. You have chosen hypnosis as the median to achieve this goal and hypnosis is a huge aid in changing your emotional attraction to food and eating permanently. Over time you have realized that hypnosis is a new positive approach- a positive approach to getting what you desire.

For the very first time in your life, you are going to initiate a positive approach towards food, eating and a healthy lifestyle. As you initiate this positive approach towards food, you are going to enjoy food, like food, eat food. You are going to make permanent positive changes in your diet. You are going to prove to your body than eating when you are physically hungry can and will satisfy all your needs, just like drinking all the water you need.

Instead of treating your appetite as an enemy or trying to kill your appetite, you are going to work within the framework of your natural reflexes, becoming a friend to your appetite, paying attention to your cravings, this is a good thing. Slim people do have appetites but they pay attention to them. Attractive people do have appetites but they pay attention to them. Hypnosis is going to make you a friend of your appetite, rather than an enemy.

Previously you have been paying attention to only half the signals from your appetite. Chiefly, the signal that says, "Eat. I am hungry." But slowly and steadily you are becoming a friend to your appetite. You are going to listen to all of what your friend's say. When it says "I am hungry," you eat. And when the hungriness disappear, and your appetite says, "I am satisfied," you take a step back. You stop way before you are full because once you feel the sensation it means that you have overeaten. You should never want this feeling again.

You are going to realise that you have not been paying a lot of attention to your appetite because your eating is not been driven by hunger but by emotions. It is always right to eat when your body says, "I am hungry." But you on the other hand have been eating even when you are not hungry. You have been eating at times out of the habit even when your the body had no biological need for food. You have been eating to satisfy your cravings and psychological needs.

You have not paid a lot of attention to your appetite when it says "I am done" or "I am satisfied". You have not paid attention to the signal "Stop eating" either. Your appetite does not need killing off but rather it needs reinforcement. Hypnosis is going to make you a friend of your appetite so you need to pay attention to the suggestions of this new friend. Tune in your body senses. If you don't follow up with your new friend, it is going to violate your normal reflexes.

Pause

It's of the utmost importance that you should eat all you physiologically need to replace your energy stores for sudden use and store your body's sugar. I am advising you to drop all the plans that you have in your mind for dieting. You have to do so. Otherwise, you are going to bring into action an old tendency for self-preservation.

This is going to damage all the favourable results that you are planning to achieve through hypnosis. You must develop this habit right now, that you are going to eat only when you need. Hypnosis is going to help you reinforce the normal feedback mechanism, the checks and balances that inform you that you are full, when you need food or when your appetite is satisfied.

Pause

Moreover how strong this hypnosis might be, it cannot overcome the basic principles for survival. And the most important principle is self-preservation. Surprisingly, your huge concern about being overweight is leading you to sporadic dieting. Which results in starvation as an outcome. Which in turn demands defence. Which in turn brings out the instinct of self-survival. This instinct is solely responsible for checking on your excess fat.

Pause

Think about yourself as a thin, desirable person, the thin, attractive and beautiful person that you are going to be soon. Very soon you are going to say the very same thing. As you begin to talk and feel like a slim, attractive and healthy person, you are going to soon become one.

Being overweight is not exactly a dietary problem rather it's an emotional problem. You must settle right now at this point to give up on dieting forever. You are going to make a habit to eat only when you are physically hungry and when your body needs energy. Paying attention to your appetite, paying attention to your reflexes, paying attention to feed-back patterns, reinforcing the sensation. You may lose slowly and steadily at the start. The excess fat is going to burn with time. You are going to be slim, beautiful and attractive.

You are going to feel wonderful and desirable in every way. The two words diet and dieting will be removed from your mind and all the plans that you have for dieting and you want to follow them up are going to be removed from your mind thoroughly. Dieting brings about hungriness and makes you give up on food, which in place starts the anxiety about deficiency which brings forth the feeling of self-preservation. So you are going to be through with dieting, through with dieting forever.

Pause

Through hypnosis, you are going to restore normal reflexes that will make you content and fulfilled and will bring the wonderful feeling of well-being. The word dieting is not a positive word and it threatens you with the denial of food and even death. On another hand, hypnosis is a positive word and it makes you happy, prosperous and relaxed. Diets fail whereas hypnosis succeeds.

Pause

Diets get you starvation which eventually leads to overeating which brings heftiness. Hypnosis on the other side brings gratification which leads to peace and brings about a healthy, desirable, beautiful body, a relaxed mind and a satiated spirit. The old perception of dieting is now completely removed from your mind as of now and you have realised that the actual answer is in restoring normal reflexes.

Pause

You are going to concentrate on it, taking seriously every suggestion that I am giving you, hypnosis is a positive approach. Hypnotic suggestions which you will receive from me will rapidly bring about a transformation which is of utmost importance to ensure a permanently fit, strong, desirable body which you desire.

Pause

EACH TIME WHEN YOU CRAVE TO EAT OR DRINK SOMETHING THAT YOU KNOW IS NOT GOOD FOR YOUR BODY, YOU ARE GOING TO SAY"NO" AND YOU HAVE YO STICK BY IT BECAUSE THE REWARD YOU ARE GETTING FOR THIS IS VERY IMPORTANT TO YOU THAN. EATING THE WRONG FOOD FOR THE SAKE OF YOUR CRAVINGS.

Stop Overanalyzing

Now, as we begin this session, I want you to relax and let go of your analytical mind. Let go of any desire to assess or judge.

Let your mind feel light and easy like a boat floating in calm waters.

And as you relax, I want you to let go of the need to assess this session or the words you are listening to or the need to judge me.

Let your mind feel free and allow it to just absorb all the thoughts and sounds without any judgement.

Let go of the need to overthink or over analyse.

Now observe how your body is beginning to relax.

Notice how a sense of calmness is slowly taking over your mind and body.

In this calm state of mind, you are about to take a new direction in how you see things. You will appreciate things, situations and people for what they are or as they are.

You will not spend your precious time over scrutinizing every little detail.

From here on, you are starting afresh. You are beginning to see the world in a different light. A world where you don't spend time over assessing, but instead, you are able to see everything exactly as it is without passing judgements.

Your thoughts will be positive.

You will no longer spend time debating options in your head.

You will be able to make decisions quickly and effectively.

You will be able to decide on the spot, and you will be confident in making these decisions.

You have realized that most often your first decision has always been right, and that's why you now have more trust in your gut feeling, more trust in your instincts.

The old you would have taken ten minutes to decide, but the new you is able to make these decisions instantly without any hesitation, and that's because the new you is a lot more confident. The new you has a lot more faith in your ability to make the right decisions.

You have realized that since you have stopped over analysing, you have begun to trust yourself more, and you are a lot more positive.

And you have a lot more time on hand, and you have learned to use this precious time appreciating the world all around you.

In the past you engrossed yourself with every little detail, most of it unnecessarily, and because of over analysing these tiny details, you actually missed out on the big picture.

But now that you have made this immense positive mind shift, and you are able to notice even the subtlest of wonders all around you.

Now I want you to imagine yourself in some of these situations in the past where you spent a lot of time over analysing, and notice how the answer was right under your nose all along.

This is because you are now able to channelize your thoughts and energies effectively which in return allows you to see the bigger picture at once.

And this has also helped you find a lot of free time for yourself because you no longer waste your time debating a situation inside your head.

When faced with a situation which requires you to make a decision, you are able to quickly make an effective decision because you have a lot more confidence in yourself.

The time when your friends and family called you an over thinker is a thing of the past.

Now, people enjoy coming to you for advice because you are such a good decision maker.

You are always confident and you are able make quick and effective decisions no matter what the situation.

Now, picture yourself in this new avatar, and notice how accomplished you feel. You are able to see the positive side because you are happy and confident. You enjoy life a lot more. You feel proud of yourself.

Your life has changed positively for good. Your life now seems a lot more simple, and you now feel a lot more content and relaxed.

So, go ahead and continue to relax and let your mind and body feel at ease.

Allow yourself to feel and enjoy all the wonderful things all around you.

Stop Eating Carbs

As you continue to relax deeply, allow your mind to feel the calmness all around you.

And in this deep, relaxed state of mind, I would like you to imagine a table filled with all the carbohydrates you used to once enjoy eating.

Now, I want you to rate these carbohydrates on a scale of one to ten, one being the least acceptable, and ten being highly acceptable and delicious.

So take a few moments, and play close attention to the food on the table, and think about how you would rate these carbohydrates.

Let's say you rate it an eight on the scale for now.

But then as you begin to observe it closely, you realize how bad these food choices are for your health, and how it massively jeopardises your goal in achieving that ideal body, and so you are slowly beginning to realize that you should rate it a seven now.

Now, as you continue to observe the food, you notice how it slowly begins to lose its initial appeal.

These foods are all processed foods which carry a lot of preservatives and many other unhealthy substances which you know isn't good for you at all, and so you are now thinking of rating it a six instead.

The more you look at the food, the more you realise all the disadvantages that come with it, and the more disadvantages you see, the lower you rate it.

So, now as the food begins to lose its charm even further, it looks to be more like a five, and you no longer find it as appealing.

Now, as we go deeper, I want you to pay closer attention to how these foods slowly lose their freshness.

What initially looked crunchy and delicious, now looks soggy and not as enticing as your first impression.

With that in mind, you now rate these carbohydrates a four.

As we go deeper into a relaxed state, you are now able to assess every single detail, and you are able to notice each and every food stuff individually, and you notice all the unhealthy ingredients that will ruin your health and all your hard work, and you begin to feel a sense of disgust taking over you.

And so, you now rate it a three.

The food now begins to emit a really bad smell, and you feel absolutely disgusted.

You can't imagine how you used to once eat these things.

As you continue further, you notice the food beginning to slowly turn rotten, and you notice all the flies gathering around it, and you feel sick looking at it, and so you rate it a two.

This no longer looks like food anymore. It looks disgusting and moldy.

Now, when I call out the next number, all those carbohydrates will look so repelling. It will look just like those creepy insects you cannot bear to see.

You push the table away from you because you can no longer stand the smell or sight of this food.

You are so disgusted by the entire experience that you can no longer find these carbohydrates appealing anymore.

From now on, you will never see these carbohydrates as food.

It will always remind you of this experience, and you will always picture it as unacceptable lumps of mold.

Any time you try, your body will immediately reject it.

Now I want you to breathe in deeply, and you inhale slowly, I want you to feel the confidence and relaxation take over your body.

And as you exhale, I want you to feel all the cravings for carbohydrates being slowly released from your mind and body.

Take a few more deep breaths, and let your body relax deeply.

As you continue to breathe effortlessly, you realise you no longer have any desire for carbohydrates.

You are free from these cravings for good. They are now a thing of the past.

So with that I would like you to relax deeply, and realize that everything is going to be just fine.

Manage Your Anxiety Better

One of the best ways to manage anxiety and to beat it, is to gain control over it by regaining control over yourself. With the help of this session today, you will be able to achieve more control and anxiety will no longer be a problem in your life, making you feel happier and more confident.

There is a part of you that is amazingly creative and imaginative... I would like this part of you to help you visualize yourself in a wonderful place which is free of anxiety... this could be a place that you have been to before... or a place that your mind would like to create for you now. Just take a deep breath and let your mind whisk you away to this beautiful anxiety-free place.

You can see this place so clearly in your mind that it feels very real and you are in it... This is a place where you have the liberty to surround yourself with the things or people or activities that are fun and bring you joy... putting your mind at ease... taking away all the stress as you find yourself surrounded by such joy... Take your time and build this place in your mind...

Pause

As you find yourself feeling more and more comfortable in this place... take a deep breath in through the nose, filling up your lungs slowly and gently, and as you slowly exhale through the mouth you start to feel more and more at ease... That's right... Take another deep breath in, slowly, and find yourself relaxing twice as much as you exhale... Take one more deep breath in, this time feeling so heavily relaxed, and the relaxation doubles as you breathe out... Let this relaxation sink even deeper as you return to a regular pace of breath.

Pause

You are filled with joy and wonder and peace as you enjoy your time in this place... With each passing moment these wonderful feelings grow stronger and deeper... You feel safe and relaxed... soak in every detail of this place and let it etch itself into your memory very clearly.

Pause

At any time in the future when you find yourself in a situation that makes you feel anxious or stressed, simply close your eyes, take a few deep breaths, and let your mind bring you back to this place where you feel wonder and joy and free from all worries.

And now, let us try this once here and now to make sure you have a good grasp of it.

So, take a moment here to recall any situation that caused you to feel anxious in the past.

Simply take a deep breath in now and let yourself be taken to your special place… with each breath allow yourself to feel more and more relaxed and soak in the joy of this wonderful place… and upon your next breath you feel completely at ease… free from all anxiety… feeling great and wonderful.

Become More Confident

And now that your body is so deeply relaxed, you can feel this heavy relaxation settling into every nook and corner of your body... Helping you release all tension and stress... your mind is completely at ease... You have taken a monumental step towards helping yourself and that makes you feel more confident about yourself.

You have a newfound strength within you... it continues to grow with each passing moment... this inner strength provides you with the motivation to face all challenges head-on and overcome them with flying colours... you feel stronger and more motivated to overcome the obstacles on your path to joy and a happy social life... you find yourself facing these challenges and overcoming all obstacles with a calm mind and clear thinking at all times... this calm and confident state of mind is the key to unlocking all your potential.

Pause

And now with so much confidence and calmness and strength within you, you can feel your self-respect growing... your self-respect and self-confidence will continue to grow manifold with each passing day.

With this confidence in yourself and clarity in your mind, you are able to replace every bit of helplessness that you felt in the past, being replaced by greater confidence and self-control... You are a happier person with a zest to live life to the fullest... you have a positive outlook towards life and all that comes with it... and this is helping you find success in all your endeavours... You have all the skills and abilities needed for such success within you.

Pause

You can now see clearly how the unhappiness in relationships is a byproduct of judging yourself as well as others, and holding yourself back by building too many walls... You know now that love comes naturally in your relationships with others when you are able to completely and unconditionally love and accept yourself first... You have no need to approve the actions or appearance of other people in order for you to be able to love them... You find your love for yourself growing and with it the unconditional acceptance of others... You feel more loved and more loving... you feel more confident and content.

Script for Ego Strengthening and Success

Take a deep breath and allow yourself to soak in this heavy sense of relaxation taking over you... Just sit back and let it sink in... That's right.

And now I would like you to take a moment here to reflect on the greatness within you... recall what a truly wonderful person you are... Recall all the amazing achievements you have had through all these years owing to your natural tendency to learn and grow... All of these wonderful capabilities help you grow stronger each day... I would like you to focus on the ease with which you are able to achieve success... right from the moment you were born to now... you have been built for success and it is evident from your countless achievements... right from the day you began to crawl... to the day you learned to walk... maybe even ride a bike or drive a car...

Recall how when you were born, you didn't know how to speak right away... but you learnt how to speak in a very short span of time... to now when weaving words into meaningful expressions is a second nature to you... These abilities help you express yourself gently and clearly... all this comes naturally to you as you were born to succeed.

Call to mind all of those early school years and the challenges you faced during that time... think of how you faced each challenge and emerged with new skills and achievements each time... Think of all the subjects you have been able to master in all these years... building each success on the strong foundation of the previous successes...

Take a moment to take pride in yourself for having grown by facing so many different stages and challenges in life... how you have learnt so many valuable life lessons... forging friendships... holding jobs... seeking new experiences in life... and how wonderfully you have built a life that is interesting and immensely satisfying.

And just like you have so effortlessly sailed through life and succeeded at each step... you already know that you will continue to find success in the present and the future... this is something that you are built for... something that comes naturally to you... and it will continue and grow with each passing day, throughout your life... You will continue to succeed because you are confident in yourself and your abilities... you are in control of your life... whatever you put your mind to, you achieve... you are able to fulfil your desires because you are a remarkable human being with a remarkable mind and abilities... far greater than you can imagine... These abilities help broaden your horizons and tap into your immense potential and creativity... So allow your creativity and your mind to open up to greatness because you deserve it.

You are so deeply relaxed... you are now open and willing to accept the rewarding suggestions that I am about to give.

Even if you find the thoughts in your mind drifting or fading away, know that your subconscious mind is active and attentive... it is going to note down every positive suggestion that I have to offer... you are deeply relaxed and enjoying this process.

You are ready to face any challenge that life throws at you...

You are confident and you are strong...

You are full of joy and energy...

You are looking forward to trying new things...

With each breath you take, you are feeling better and better...

You are strong and wise...

You can achieve everything you set your mind to...

You are enjoying life to the fullest...

You can see the goodness in the world and the people around you.

Boost Happiness

Allow yourself to relax further and further... deeper and deeper... and as you allow this relaxation to sink in deeply, take a moment to visualise a place and a time when you felt really happy... such a time when you laughed out loud... A time when you, and everyone around you felt happy.

I would like you to imagine that you are on a camping trip... accompanied by your friends and family you are taking a hike... It is a warm and bright sunny day... there is a cool and comforting breeze grazing past you... You look around and notice all the tall trees and their vibrant shades of green and brown... you can smell the fragrance of pine as you breathe in... You can hear the birds happily chirping in these woods... You can notice the squirrels whizzing up and down the trees... You can even notice the sound of water falling on rocks from a tall waterfall a few meters ahead of you... you can spot the rainbow in the mist from the waterfall... You can even see little butterflies flying among the tiny colourful flowers amidst the grass.

You take a pause from walking and decide to set up camp here... You spread a white and red chequered mat on the forest floor and everyone sits down... your friends begin to open up the food packets and suddenly the air around is full of the fragrance of your favourite food... You sit here sharing a meal after hours of hiking in the woods with your near and dear ones... you share food and laughter... you are enjoying the company.

After finishing your meal, you head to the stream to drink some fresh and clean water... as you dip your hand in, you feel the cool freshness of the water filling you up with more joy... You spontaneously splash your friends with some of the water... and they all begin to join the fun... splashing water and wading in the pool like little carefree kids... feeling happy and content.

After a while you all decide to sit by the side of the mountain... gazing at the horizon in the distance as the sun begins to set over the valley... the sky is lit up in vibrant colours... various shades of red, orange, even purple... Looking at this scene brings you immense joy and satisfaction... you feel happy and satisfied.

You are so relaxed and full of joy... your mind is now open and accepting of the positive suggestion I am about to give... Your subconscious mind is still active and taking note of these suggestions...

You are in charge of how you feel, and you choose to feel happy...

You forgive yourself for not being perfect...

You are worthy of all the good things in life...

You see struggles as opportunities to grow and learn...

You accept yourself unconditionally and completely...

You are stronger than you know...

You love yourself and you are able to let go of anything that does not serve you...

Affirmations

1. Losing weight is a natural process for you. (7 seconds pause)

2. You are happily achieving your goals of losing weight. (7 seconds pause)

3. Every day you are losing weight (7 seconds pause)

4. You love to work out regularly. (7 seconds pause)

5. You are consuming food that contributes to your health. (7 seconds pause)

6. You eat only when you feel like eating. (7 seconds pause)

7. You can now clearly see yourself at your ideal weight. (7 seconds pause)

8. You love the flavours of healthy food. (7 seconds pause)

9. You have control over how much eat. (7 seconds pause)

10. You are enjoying workouts, it makes you feel confident.

11. Through exercise you are getting slimmer and stronger every day. (7 seconds pause)

12. You can easily reach and maintain your goal weight. (7 seconds pause)

13. You love and care for your body (7 seconds pause)

14. You deserve a slim, beautiful and desirable body. (7 seconds pause)

15. You have developed a healthy eating habit. (7 seconds pause)

16. You are getting fitter every day. (7 seconds pause)

17. You look great. (7 seconds pause)

18. You do whatever it takes to be healthy. (7 seconds pause)

19. You have happily redefined success. (7 seconds pause)

20. You choose to exercise every day. (7 seconds pause)

21. You want to eat food that makes you feel good about yourself. (7 seconds pause)

22. You are responsible for your health. (7 seconds pause)

23. You love your body. (7 seconds pause)

24. You are patient with creating a better body. (7 seconds pause)

25. You are happily exercising every morning so that you can very easily reach your goal weight. (7 seconds pause)

26. You have changed your eating habit from unhealthy to healthy. (7 seconds pause)

27. You are happy with every part you do to lose weight. (7 seconds pause)

28. Every day you are getting fitter and stronger. (7 seconds pause)

29. You are in the process of developing a healthy body. (7 seconds pause)

30. You are developing vibrant health. (7 seconds pause)

31. You are creating a body that you like and enjoy. (7 seconds pause)

Positive Affirmations For Losing Weight. (7 seconds pause)

1. Your lifestyle eating patterns are changing your body. (7 seconds pause)

2. You have lost 10 pounds in 4 weeks and you are very excited to meet your lady friend. (7 seconds pause)

3. You have a toned stomach. (7 seconds pause)

4. You like to make your own choices about food. (7 seconds pause)

5. You are happily weighing 20 pounds less. (7 seconds pause)

6. You love walking 3-4 times a week and you like to do toning exercise 3 times a week. (7 seconds pause)

7. You drink 8 glasses of water every day. (7 seconds pause)

8. You eat fruits, vegetables, chicken and fish regularly. (7 seconds pause)

9. You are using mental, emotional and spiritual skills for success. You are willing the change! (7 seconds pause)

10. You are willing to create new thoughts and ideas about yourself and your body. (7 seconds pause)

11. You love and appreciate your body. (7 seconds pause)

12. It is exciting to discover new ideas and different foods for weight loss. (7 seconds pause)

13. You have a very beautiful weight loss success story that you are willing to share with everyone out there. (7 seconds pause)

14. You are delighted and extremely happy to be at your goal weight. (7 seconds pause)

15. It is easy for you to follow a healthy diet plan with time. (7 seconds pause)

16. You choose to embrace thoughts of confidence in your ability to make some serious positive changes in your life. (7 seconds pause)

17. It feels great to move your body and workouts are fun. (7 seconds pause)

18. You use deep breathing techniques which helps you to handle stress and makes your body feel relaxed. (7 seconds pause)

19. You are a beautiful person inside out. (7 seconds pause)

20. You deserve to be at your goal weight. (7 seconds pause)

21. You are a healthy and lovable person. You deserve all the love. It is safe for you to lose weight. (7 seconds pause)

22. You are a strong presence in the world at my lower weight. (7 seconds pause)

23. You release the need to criticise your body. (7 seconds pause)

24. You accept and enjoy your sexuality. It is completely Ok to feel sensuous. (7 seconds pause)

25. Your metabolism is very good. (7 seconds pause)

26. You maintain your body with optimal health. (7 seconds pause)

1You believe in your ability to love and appreciate yourself for who you are. (7 seconds pause)

2. You set yourself free from all the guilt and negative thoughts about the food that you chose in the past. (12 seconds pause)

3.Every day you are working out and taking care of your body. (7 seconds pause)

4. Healing is happening in both your body and mind. (7 seconds pause)

5. Every time you breathe in, fresh energy fills your entire body with positivity and every time you exhale, all toxins and fats leaves your body. (12 seconds pause)

6. Your health is improving every day and so is your body. (7 seconds pause)

7. Every thing that you consume heals and nourishes your body, which helps you reach your goal weight. (7 seconds pause)

8. You are moving closer and closer to your goal weight with each passing day. (7 seconds pause)

9. You are so happy with your weight. (7 seconds pause)

10. You feel like you can do this you are doing this, your body is losing weight every day. (7 seconds pause)

11. You are letting go of all the guilt that you hold around food. (7 seconds pause)

12. Eating healthy food helps your body get all the nutrients it needs to be in the best shape and size. (7 seconds pause)

13. You are moving more closer to your ideal weight with each passing day. (7 seconds pause)

14. You feel the desire for fat-rich foods dissolving. (7 seconds pause)

15. You have a strong urge to eat only foods rich in nutrients, not unhealthy processed foods. (7 seconds pause)

16. You are becoming the best version of yourself, you are even thriving to become better than ever. You are going to lose weight because you want to, and you have the power to do this. (17 seconds pause)

17. Your body is your temple and you are taking care of it by eating healthy and in right amount. (7 seconds pause)

18. You are aware that your metabolism is working in the right direction and is helping you in gaining your optimal weight. (7 seconds pause)

19. You are maintaining your desired weight. (7 seconds pause)

20. You have the power to control your weight through healthy eating and exercising regularly. (12 seconds pause)

21. You are grateful to your body for all the things it does. (7 seconds pause)

22. Every cell in your body is working great and so are you. (7 seconds pause)

23. You feel that your body is losing weight every second of the day. (7 seconds pause)

24. You chew your food in the right way so that your body can digest it and take out all the desired nutrients to lose weight. (12 seconds pause)

25. You believe in your ability to change habits and create new healthy habits. (7 seconds pause)

26. You no longer feel the urge to stuff your stomach with food, now you can easily resist temptations. (7 seconds pause)

27. You enjoy life by staying healthy and eating healthy. (7 seconds pause)

28. You are capable enough to achieve your ideal weight. (7 seconds pause)

29. You accept your body however it is and you are constantly working on it to improve it. (7 seconds pause)

30. You very nicely understand that unhealthy food is not going to help you lose weight, so you should eat only healthy food rich in nutrients. (7 seconds pause)

31. Your metabolism rate is at its optimum level and it is constantly helping you to reach your ideal weight. (7 seconds pause)

32. You are a confident person whom everyone loves and respects. (7 seconds pause)

33. You are an unique person and you deserve all ta respect that you are getting. (7 seconds pause)

34. You accept and love yourself for who you are. (7 seconds pause)

35. To you it does not matter what other people have to say. What matters to you is how you react and what you believe in. (7 seconds pause)

36. Your mind is filled with positive thoughts and you do not entertain any negativity. (7 seconds pause)

37. You breathe in relaxation and breathe out stress. (7 seconds pause)

38. You respect yourself and so do others around you. (7 seconds pause)

39. You accept yourself the way you are and you are happy with your life. (7 seconds pause)

40. You accept every single thing that you have in your mind and you live in absolute joy. (7 seconds pause)

41. You feel excited about challenges that life has to offer and you happily go through them without any anxiety and guilt. (12 seconds pause)

42. You replace "I should" "I have to" "I must" with "I choose". (7 seconds pause)

43. You have full trust in yourself and you know that you are a worthy person and that is why everyone respects you. (7 seconds pause)

44..Meeting new people is becoming easier for you. You can make new friends without feeling anxious. (7 seconds pause)

45. You pay attention to both your qualities and defects and you thrive to improve them. (7 seconds pause)

46.You are a very attentive person and you do not quit to do anything even when you feel challenged or wronged. (12 seconds pause)

47. You are kind, caring and loyal to the people around you. You inhale self-confidence and exhale fear and anxiety. (7 seconds pause)

48.You have integrity and you are a very reliable person, you do exactly what is said to you and everyone can trust you. (7 seconds pause)

49. You trust and believe in yourself and let go of every the negative thought that crosses your mind. (7 seconds pause)

50. Being alive makes you happy and excited. (7 seconds pause)

51. Being yourself is good and rewarding and you always perceive challenges as opportunities to do better and better. (7 seconds pause)

52. You deserve all that you want. You release any need of suffering and you can feel happiness, confidence and love getting into your mind, body and soul. (7 seconds pause)

53. You are enthusiastic and energetic and confidence is an important part of your nature. (7 seconds pause)

54. You are healthy, beautiful and attractive and you appreciate both inner and outer beauty. (7 seconds pause)

55. You thrive on absolute self-confidence. Your life is beautiful and you enjoy every single second of it. (7 seconds pause)

56. You never compare yourself to others as you know you are perfect the way you are. (7 seconds pause)

57. When you inhale confidence fills your entire body and when you exhale all the guilt and shyness gets out of your body automatically. (7 seconds pause)

58. You accept yourself however you are and you are getting better and better with time. (7 seconds pause)

59. You are a person who accepts new challenges and opportunities. (7 seconds pause)

60. Opportunity is a challenge for you which you accept wholeheartedly. (7 seconds pause)

61. Affirmations for weight loss. (7 seconds pause)

62.You are lively, energetic and high on energy. (7 seconds pause)

63.Your next meal is so bland that your life seems interesting. (7 seconds pause)

64. Your body is against unhealthy fatty foods, it only demands healthy, fresh and real food! (7 seconds pause)

65. Binge eating won't appeal you or your goals. (7 seconds pause)

66. You calculate before you surrender to cravings. (7 seconds pause)

67. You chose to pamper your body today. (7 seconds pause)

68. You are-associated with your higher self. (7 seconds pause)

69. You are a sportsperson and you are competent and proficient of great disciplines. (7 seconds pause).

70. You have mastery in self-control before indulging into momentary impulses. (7 seconds pause)

71. You dare to accept what works for you and change accordingly. (7 seconds pause)

72. You have conquered over momentary impulse and choose food with sincerity. (7 seconds pause).

73. You are determined enough and hustle hard each day to reach your goal weight. (7 seconds pause)

74. Every time you suppress your cravings you boost your self-mastery. (7 seconds pause)

75. You are on a journey and you don't like to compare it with others. (7 seconds pause)

76. You are mature enough to handle all the wounds that life has to offer. (7 seconds pause)

77. You are energetic, vibrant and full of energy. (7 seconds pause)

78. You allow your journey to be unique. (7 seconds pause)

79. Maintaning your ideal weight is not a big deal. (7 seconds pause)

80. You live, eat and listen with all your heart. (7 seconds pause)

81. You understand that your thoughts are mere emotions and are not real.

82. You believe in at the moment things. (7 seconds pause)

83. You turn the daily tasks into knowledgeable moments. (7 seconds pause)

84. You dare to challenge existing ideas. (7 seconds pause)

85. You are at peace with your past. (7 seconds pause)

86. You go outdoors to grasp at the beauty of nature. (7 seconds pause)

87. You enjoy every bit of your meal. (7 seconds pause)

88. Your stamina and energy increase with every breathe you take. (7 seconds pause)

89. You think twice before eating something. (7 seconds pause)

90. Your body gets nourished with each and everything that you put in your mouth. (7 seconds pause)

91. There is a new ray of hope each day. (7 seconds pause)

92. Your desire to live longer is more than your cravings. (7 seconds pause)

93. Your confidence lies in feeling healthy, fresh and energetic. (7 seconds pause)

94. You enjoy feeling your heartbeat. (7 seconds pause)

95. You think before surrendering to your cravings. (7 seconds pause)

96. Your healthy habits are a part and parcel of your life.(7 seconds pause)

97. You have the realization that thoughts are ideas that need to be controlled. (7 seconds pause)

98. Your will power is beyond any plating, food or goal. (7 seconds pause)

99. You chose to cure, nourish and pamper your mind and body today. (7 seconds pause)

100. You are creating a life of prosperity. (7 seconds pause)

101. Your goals in life allow you to live every moment. (7 seconds pause)

102. You are moving ahead every single day. (7 seconds pause)

103. You crave fresh fruits and vegetables to feel rejuvenated. (7 seconds pause)

104. You chew meals very carefully so that it gets digested and helps you to reach your goal weight. (7 seconds pause)
105. Your metabolism is with you on this journey from fat to fit. (7 seconds pause)
106. You let the guilt go away when you are around food. (7 seconds pause)
107. You breathe in peace and breathe out tension. (7 seconds pause)
108. You acknowledge your journey to be unique and do not compare with others. (7 seconds pause)
109. You drink a lot of water to elate your mood and metabolism. (7 seconds pause)
110. Your desire to reach your ideal weight has made your food choices to be consistent. (7 seconds pause)
111. You are willing to explore new things every day. (7 seconds pause)

Affirmations for Positivity and Success

1. You are in charge of how you feel… And you choose to feel happy. (7 seconds pause)
2. Your anxiety has no control over your decision-making power (7 seconds pause)
3. You are worthy of all the good things in life (7 seconds pause)
4. At this moment, right now, you are choosing happiness (7 seconds pause)
5. With every breath you take, you inhale confidence and exhale fear (7 seconds pause)
6. Even if you suffer a setback, you do not get stuck, you soldier on (7 seconds pause)
7. You forgive yourself for not being perfect (7 seconds pause)
8. You are learning to support and encourage your best self (7 seconds pause)
9. You view struggles as opportunities for growth and learning (7 seconds pause)
10. Your past has no power over you (7 seconds pause)
11. You have survived these feelings before, you can do it again (7 seconds pause)
12. You accept yourself completely and unconditionally (7 seconds pause)
13. You are choosing to stop apologising for being your true self (7 seconds pause)
14. Your life has meaning and purpose (7 seconds pause)
15. You are stronger than you know (7 seconds pause)
16. You always give yourself space to grow and learn (7 seconds pause)
17. You find beauty in everything, everyday (7 seconds pause)
18. You are not alone in your struggle (7 seconds pause)
19. This is temporary and it will pass (7 seconds pause)
20. You allow yourself to feel every emotion but not linger in them (7 seconds pause)
21. You care for yourself and self-care is not selfish (7 seconds pause)
22. You allow yourself to seek help and lean on others when you feel out of depth (7 seconds pause)
23. You will never have to go through today again (7 seconds pause)
24. You are ready to let go of everything that no longer serves you (7 seconds pause)
25. You are greater than your anxiety (7 seconds pause)
26. With every breath you take, you feel calmer and more at ease (7 seconds pause)
27. You are able to accept the things you cannot change (7 seconds pause)
28. Not everything weighing you down is yours to carry, let go (7 seconds pause)
29. These feelings won't last (7 seconds pause)
30. You are kinder to yourself (7 seconds pause)
31. You deserve to be gentle with yourself (7 seconds pause)
32. You talk to yourself like you talk to the ones you love (7 seconds pause)
33. One bad day does not mean yours is a bad life (7 seconds pause)
34. You will breathe deeply and slowly (7 seconds pause)

35. You choose to focus on today, one hour at a time, one moment at a time (7 seconds pause)
36. You are letting go of toxicity in your thoughts, feelings, and actions (7 seconds pause)
37. You are letting go of negative energy (7 seconds pause)
38. You control your thoughts, your thoughts have no control over you (7 seconds pause)
39. Tomorrow is a brand new day (7 seconds pause)
40. You live your life with authenticity and courage (7 seconds pause)
41. You are proud of yourself for trying (7 seconds pause)
42. You are resilient and strong (7 seconds pause)
43. You allow yourself to feel this way (7 seconds pause)
44. You are proud that you are not what you used to be anymore (7 seconds pause)
45. You are still healing and it is okay (7 seconds pause)
46. You can feel anxious and still be able to deal with this situation (7 seconds pause)
47. You are successful (7 seconds pause)
48. You allow yourself to feel scared but the fear does not control you (7 seconds pause)
49. You love yourself deeply and unconditionally (7 seconds pause)
50. You are an achiever (7 seconds pause)

CPSIA information can be obtained
at www.ICGtesting.com
Printed in the USA
LVHW060203240622
722036LV00006B/99